Nature's Viral Defenders

Harnessing the Power of Herbal Antivirals

Olivia Grant

Table of Contents

INTRODUCTION

Detailed overview of the viral challenges of today and the importance of herbal antivirals

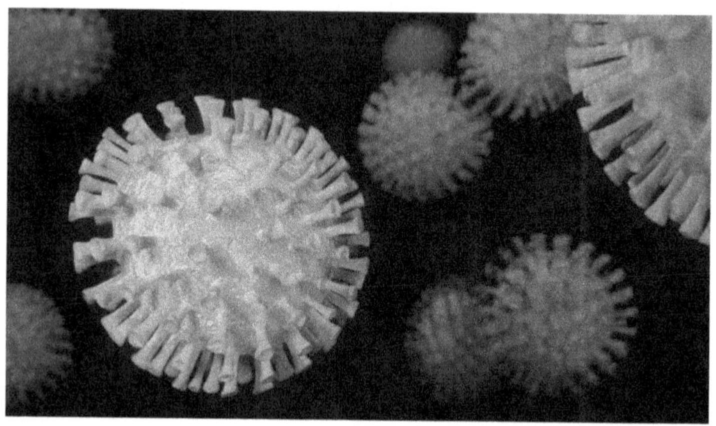

Since the beginning of recorded history, the possibility of contracting a viral infection has been one of humanity's primary worries. Since the discovery of novel viruses and the occurrence of pandemics on a global scale, this probability has only grown. During the course of the last ten years, we have seen various outbreaks of potentially fatal viruses, including Ebola, Zika, and COVID-19. These epidemics have caused widespread alarm and economic damage, underscoring the need for comprehensive ways to prevent and cure infectious diseases caused by viruses.

Even though there have been great advancements in the treatment of viral infections by modern medicine, there is an increasing interest in employing natural therapies such as herbal antivirals to support the immune system and create resilience against viral threats. This section provides a detailed overview of the current viral threats and the significance of herbal antivirals in the fight against viral infections.

Globally, humanity is currently confronting a number of viral threats, some of which have already caused substantial damage to public health as well as the economy of the entire world. The following are some of the most serious viral dangers that the world is now facing:

COVID-19 is a newly discovered coronavirus that first appeared in Wuhan, China, in December of 2019. It swiftly dispersed throughout the world, resulting in a pandemic on a worldwide scale. There have been almost 200 million confirmed cases of COVID-19, and there have been 4 million deaths as of August 2021. This has led to severe morbidity and mortality. The epidemic has also had a huge impact on the economy, with several countries suffering from recession and job loss as a direct result.

Influenza, more often known as the flu, is a contagious viral illness that affects millions of people annually. The flu can cause severe morbidity and mortality, especially in susceptible populations including the elderly and those who already have preexisting medical issues. While vaccines are available for influenza, the virus mutates rapidly, making it difficult to develop effective vaccines.

HIV/AIDS is a viral infection that affects the immune system. While substantial progress has been made in treating and preventing HIV/AIDS, the virus remains a significant worldwide health issue, particularly in low- and middle-income nations.

Both hepatitis B and hepatitis C are infectious diseases that impact the liver. Especially in people who already have chronic illnesses, these viruses can cause severe morbidity and mortality. There are vaccines available for hepatitis B, but there is currently no treatment or prevention for hepatitis C.

Traditional treatments have a number of drawbacks, especially in light of the substantial advancements that have been made in the treatment of viral infections by contemporary medicine. Antiviral therapy may be prohibitively expensive, may cause serious adverse effects, and may lead to the evolution of viruses that are resistant to therapeutic treatment. In addition, there is a rising concern regarding the misuse of antiviral drugs and antibiotics, which might result in the evolution of infections that are resistant to the effects of pharmacological treatment.

Supporting the immune system in a natural and holistic way while also preventing viral infections can be achieved through the use of herbal antivirals. Antiviral qualities have been observed in traditional herbal treatments, which have a long history of use and have been proved to be effective against a number of diseases. When it comes to the fight against viral infections, employing herbal antivirals can provide a number of benefits, including the following:

Supporting the immune system in a natural and holistic way while also preventing viral infections can be achieved through the use of herbal antivirals. Herbal therapies, in contrast to conventional pharmaceuticals, are obtained from natural sources and have a lower potential for adverse effects. They can also be used in conjunction with other natural treatments, such as adjustments to one's food and way of life, in order to provide an even higher level of immune system support.

There are a number of plants and herbs that have been identified as having substantial antiviral effects. These medicinal plants have properties that can stop the reproduction of viruses and stop the spread of viral diseases. Elderberry, echinacea, garlic, licorice root, and ginger are among the most powerful antivirals that may be obtained from plants.

Elderberry, for example, has been shown to have significant antiviral properties, particularly against influenza viruses. Echinacea is yet another herb that research has revealed to possess antiviral properties and that has the potential to treat a wide range of viral diseases. The antiviral qualities of garlic have been known for years, but only recently have they been verified by scientific research. Garlic has been used for millennia to both prevent and treat infections.

The immune system can be strengthened by the use of herbal antivirals, which in turn makes it more efficient in warding off viral diseases. It has been demonstrated that certain herbs, including astragalus, ginseng, and reishi mushrooms, can strengthen the immune system and boost its ability to fight off viral infections. Herbal antivirals are able to do this by strengthening the immune system, which in turn helps prevent viral infections from taking hold and lessens the intensity of their symptoms.

Herbal antivirals are often more cost-effective than traditional antiviral medications. Numerous herbal treatments are simple to prepare at home with components that are readily available, which makes them available to a larger number of individuals. This can be particularly important in low- and middle-income countries, where access to traditional antiviral medications may be limited.

Herbal antivirals have fewer side effects than traditional antiviral medications. It is possible for certain herbs to induce modest adverse effects such as stomach distress; but, in general, the adverse effects caused by herbs are much less severe than those caused by conventional drugs. Because of this, herbal remedies are a more secure choice than conventional medicines for people who could be allergic to conventional drugs or have preexisting health concerns.

In conclusion, the globe is currently confronting a number of viral dangers, the most prominent of which being COVID-19, influenza, HIV/AIDS, and both hepatitis B and C. Even though there have been great advancements in the treatment of viral infections by modern medicine, there is a growing interest in the utilization of natural therapies such as herbal antivirals to support the immune system and create resilience against viral threats. Herbal antivirals provide a method that is both natural and holistic for the treatment and prevention of viral infections. They are capable of strengthening the immune system, possess strong antiviral characteristics, and are frequently less expensive than conventional antiviral drugs. By incorporating herbal remedies into our daily routines, we can support our immune systems as well as build resilience against viral threats. In the fight against viral infections, herbal antivirals are a potentially helpful addition to our treatment options; however, they should not be used in place of conventional antiviral drugs.

Overview of the book's contents and purpose

Throughout the course of human history, the world has been confronted with a number of viral dangers, and it would appear that new ones emerge on an annual basis.

The COVID-19 pandemic demonstrated how susceptible we are to these dangers and how critical it is to have a robust immune system in order to ward them off and protect ourselves. Even though there have been significant advancements in the treatment and prevention of viral infections made by contemporary medicine, there is also a growing interest in the use of natural therapies such as herbal antivirals to support the immune system and create resilience against viral threats. This ebook aims to provide an overview of herbal antivirals and how they can be used to build resilience against viral threats.

The herbal antivirals and their role in the process of establishing resilience against viral threats are discussed in each of the book's six chapters, which are separated by sections within the ebook.

Introduction

The goal of the book as well as its individual chapters are summarized in the introduction. It highlights the subjects that will be discussed in the ebook and provides an explanation for the significance of herbal antivirals in the fight against viral dangers.

Chapter 1: Understanding Viruses and the Immune System

This chapter offers a fundamental introduction to viruses as well as an explanation of how viruses function. This provides an explanation of how viruses are able to enter the body, how they reproduce, and how they can lead to disease. Additionally, the immune system and its function in the battle against viruses are discussed in this chapter. It describes the ways in which the immune system detects and reacts to viral infections, as well as the ways in which it can be boosted to better combat viral dangers.

Chapter 2: Herbal Antivirals: An Overview

An overview of herbal antivirals' mechanisms of action is provided in Chapter 2. It explains what herbal antivirals are, how they are used, and why they are important in the fight against viral threats. The various types of herbal antivirals, such as herbs, roots, and mushrooms, as well as how they might be utilized to provide support for the immune system, are also discussed in this chapter.

Chapter 3: Top Herbal Antivirals for Building Resilience

The most effective herbal antivirals for boosting one's resistance to viral infections are discussed in Chapter 3. It offers in-depth information on each herbal antiviral, including its characteristics, the mechanism by which it functions, and the positive effects it has on the immune system. This chapter also discusses the numerous methods of dosing and administration that are available for each herbal antiviral, in addition to the potential adverse effects that may be brought on by their use.

Chapter 4: Herbal Antiviral Recipes and Remedies

Recipes for antiviral herbal teas, tinctures, syrups, and other types of medicines are included in Chapter 4. In addition to that, it offers dosage recommendations for each treatment as well as advice for preparing and storing herbal treatments. The chapter includes recipes for specific viral threats, as well as general immune-boosting remedies.

Chapter 5: Building Resilience with Lifestyle Changes and Natural Support

The modifications to one's way of life that can strengthen one's immune system and make one more resistant to viral assaults are discussed in Chapter 5. It offers advice on how to get a better night's sleep, handle stress better, and make exercise a regular part of your routine. The chapter also discusses a variety of different natural supports for the immune system, including essential oils and dietary supplements.

Chapter 6: Herbal Antivirals for Specific Viral Threats

The information presented in Chapter 6 gives an overview of specific viral dangers and the herbal antivirals that are most effective against them. It provides information on how to utilize herbal antivirals in combination with other therapies, as well as dose instructions and potential adverse effects associated with each one.

The conclusion highlights the main issues covered in the ebook and emphasizes the need of building resilience against viral threats. It inspires readers to take action in the direction of constructing a robust immune system and defending themselves from viral dangers. The conclusion also provides a final note of encouragement and hope for readers who may be struggling with viral infections or fears of future viral threats.

This e-book's objective is to give readers a complete understanding of herbal antivirals and the role that they play in constructing resilience against viral assaults. Readers who get a grasp of how viruses function and how the immune system reacts to them will be better equipped to protect themselves and the people they care about from contracting viral diseases.

Because of its emphasis on herbal antivirals, this book offers readers a method to strengthening their immunity and resiliency that is both natural and holistic in nature.

Readers can maintain their immune systems without the risk of experiencing the adverse effects that are associated with contemporary drugs by using natural remedies.

The book discusses changes in lifestyle as well as natural supports that might further boost the immune system. In addition to offering information on certain herbal antivirals, the book also includes this material. By making these changes, readers can not only protect themselves from viral threats but also improve their overall health and well-being.

Nature's Viral Defenders: Harnessing the Power of Herbal Antivirals is, in its entirety, a thorough guide on the utilization of natural treatments in order to support the immune system and create resistance against viral infections. Readers can take steps to protect themselves and those they care about from the effects of viral infections by first gaining an awareness of how viruses function and how the immune system reacts to viruses.

CHAPTER I

Understanding Viruses and the Immune System

Introduction to viruses and how they work

Microorganisms called viruses are infectious agents that can cause a variety of diseases in people and other living organisms. Viruses are minuscule. The genetic material, which can be either DNA or RNA, is surrounded by a protein sheath in its structure. Viruses can only reproduce themselves inside of living cells, and in order for this to happen, they require a host cell. When it comes to preventing and treating viral infections, having a solid understanding of the composition and behavior of viruses is absolutely necessary.

Viruses can range in size from 20 to 300 nanometers, demonstrating their small nature. They have a simple structure consisting of genetic material, either DNA or RNA, and a protein coat called a capsid. In addition to the capsid, certain viruses contain a lipid envelope that surrounds it.

The capsid is constructed by reoccurring protein subunits that are referred to as capsomeres. The capsid is necessary for viral replication because it guards the genetic material and prevents it from being damaged. In the event that it is present, the lipid envelope is generated from the membrane of the host cell and contains proteins that are essential for attachment to and entry into host cells.

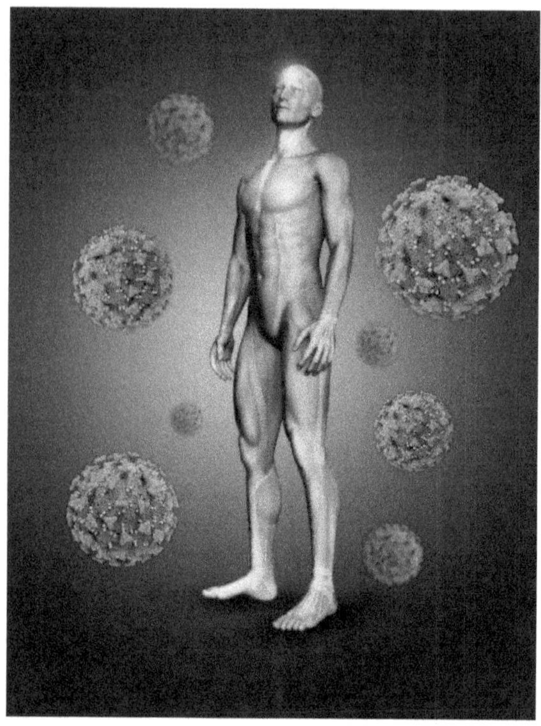

Attachment to the host cell, admission into the host cell, replication within the host cell, assembly outside of the host cell, and release from the host cell are the stages that comprise the life cycle of viruses. The following is a list of the stages that are involved in the life cycle of a virus:

The attachment of the virus to a host cell is the initial stage of the life cycle of a virus. Typically, this is accomplished through the formation of certain contacts between viral surface proteins and receptors on host cells. The attachment process is critical in determining the host range of a virus, or the types of cells and organisms that the virus can infect. There are many varieties of viruses, each of which can attach itself to a particular receptor that is located on the surface of its host cell.

Once attached, the virus enters the host cell. The means by which a virus enters a host cell might differ from virus to virus, but in general, it either includes the fusion of the viral envelope with the membrane of the host cell or the endocytosis-mediated consumption of the virus by the host cell. In some instances, the virus might not be able to enter the host cell without extra components, such as co-receptors or proteases, in order to aid its entry. Once it has entered the host cell, the virus is able to start the replication process.

Once it has entered the cell of its host, the virus will duplicate its genetic material by utilising the machinery of the host cell. The process of replication could involve the production of viral proteins and the formation of new viral particles. The replication process is critical in the life cycle of viruses, as it allows the virus to produce multiple copies of itself and continue to infect additional cells and organisms.

New viral particles are assembled inside the host cell. A full viral particle is formed when the capsid and the genetic material are brought together. The process of assembly is very precisely controlled by the virus, and many viruses use a variety of different techniques to put together their constituent parts. To assemble themselves, certain viruses may make use of the machinery of their host cells, while others may be dependent on particular viral proteins.

The discharge of new viral particles from within the host cell marks the culmination of the life cycle of the virus. This can happen when the host cell is destroyed, which is known as lysis, or it can happen when the virus bursts through the cell membrane and leaves the host cell. The process of release is an essential part of the life cycle of viruses because it paves the way for the virus to replicate and infect more cells and organisms. The mechanism of release can also influence the pathogenesis of the virus, or the severity of disease that it causes.

There are a variety of differences between the life cycles of various viruses, despite the fact that the fundamental processes in the viral life cycle are the same for all viruses. These variants have the potential to affect the pathogenesis of the virus, which refers to the severity of the disease that the virus produces.
The means by which the virus enters its host cell is one of the aspects of the life cycle of viruses that can vary significantly. To assist entry into the host cell, certain viruses may make use of a variety of receptors or co-receptors on the surface of the host cell. This can have an effect on the kinds of cells and organisms that the virus is able to infect.

The method by which the virus exits the host cell represents yet another key point of difference in the life cycle of viruses. Some viruses can cause lysis of the host cell, which can result in cell death and damage to tissue, while others can exit the host cell by budding from the cell membrane, which can be less destructive to the host cell. Some viruses can cause lysis of the host cell.

Viruses can also vary in the speed and efficiency of their replication cycle, which can influence the severity of disease that they cause. It's possible that certain viruses have a faster replication cycle, which causes the disease to be more severe, while others have a slower replication cycle, which causes the symptoms to be less severe.

The lytic cycle and the lysogenic cycle are the two most common forms of viral replication cycles.

The reproduction cycle of viruses that ultimately results in the lysis, or destruction, of the host cell is referred to as the lytic cycle. The lytic cycle is generally linked with acute viral infections, which are characterized by fast viral replication that results in substantial damage to the host cell and the tissue that surrounds it. The influenza virus and the herpes simplex virus are both examples of viruses that go through a process called the lytic cycle.

The lysogenic cycle is the stage of viral replication in which the virus integrates its genetic material into the genome of the host cell. This makes it possible for the virus to remain dormant within the host cell without inflicting any immediate damage. The lysogenic cycle is typically associated with chronic viral infections, where the virus persists in the host for an extended period without causing significant symptoms. The human papillomavirus (HPV) and the Epstein-Barr virus are both examples of viruses that go through a process called the lysogenic cycle. (EBV).

There is more than one kind of virus, each of which has the potential to trigger a different sickness in people and other living organisms. It is vital to gain an understanding of the various types of viruses in order to successfully treat and prevent viral infections.

RNA viruses are distinguished by the fact that they use RNA as their genetic material and that their replication is dependent on RNA polymerase. The influenza virus, measles virus, and hepatitis C virus are all examples of viruses that are of the RNA variety. On the basis of the organization of their genomes, RNA viruses can be further subdivided into the following categories:

RNA viruses with a positive sense of direction possess RNA genomes that are capable of being directly translated into viral proteins by the machinery present in the host cell. Examples of positive-sense RNA viruses include the SARS-CoV-2 virus, which causes COVID-19, and the hepatitis A virus.

The RNA genomes of these viruses need to be transformed into a positive-sense RNA intermediate before viral protein synthesis can take place. These viruses are classified as "negative-sense." The Ebola virus and the rabies virus are both examples of viruses that contain the negative-sense form of RNA.
Viruses that replicate using a viral RNA-dependent RNA polymerase are known as double-stranded RNA viruses. These viruses have RNA genomes that are double-stranded and replicate utilizing the enzyme. The rotavirus, which is responsible for children's severe diarrhea, is an example of a virus that has two strands of RNA.

DNA viruses employ DNA as their genetic material, and DNA-dependent DNA polymerase is the enzyme responsible for their replication. Herpes simplex virus, human papillomavirus, and varicella-zoster virus are all examples of viruses that include DNA. On the basis of the organization of their genomes, DNA viruses can be further divided into the following categories:

These viruses have DNA genomes that are single-stranded and reproduce utilizing a viral DNA-dependent DNA polymerase. Single-stranded DNA viruses are the most common type of DNA virus. One example of a virus that possesses a single strand of DNA is the parvovirus, which can lead to severe anemia in dogs.

These viruses have DNA genomes that are double-stranded and replicate using a viral DNA-dependent DNA polymerase. Adenoviruses, for instance, are examples of viruses with double-stranded DNA. Adenoviruses are known to cause respiratory infections as well as gastroenteritis.

The genetic material that retroviruses possess is RNA, but in order to multiply, they need an enzyme called reverse transcriptase to generate DNA, which is subsequently incorporated into the genome of the host cell. For instance, the human immunodeficiency virus, also known as HIV, and the human T-lymphotropic virus are both examples of retroviruses. (HTLV). The organization of a retrovirus's genome allows for additional classification of the virus, including the following:

Simple retroviruses are characterized by the presence of a single open reading frame and the generation of a single polyprotein that can be cleaved into a number of different proteins with specific functions. The Moloney murine leukemia virus and the feline leukemia virus are both examples of simple retroviruses.

Complex retroviruses are characterized by the presence of numerous open reading frames and the generation of multiple polyproteins that are subsequently cleaved into functional proteins. The human immunodeficiency virus (HIV) and the simian immunodeficiency virus are both examples of complicated retroviruses.

Adenoviruses are DNA viruses that can infect humans and cause a number of diseases, such as gastroenteritis, conjunctivitis, and respiratory infections. The genomes of adenoviruses are made up of two strands of DNA, and the replication process is catalyzed by a viral DNA-dependent DNA polymerase.

The genetic and antigenic properties of adenoviruses allow for further categorization of the virus into seven distinct species, designated by the letters A through G. There are many different diseases that can be brought on by each species, however certain species are linked to more serious ailments than others.

Herpesviruses are a class of DNA viruses that are responsible for a wide range of disorders, such as chickenpox, cold sores, and genital herpes. Herpesviruses have genomes that are made up of two strands of DNA, and in order to replicate, they need a viral DNA-dependent DNA polymerase. Herpesviruses can be further classified into three subfamilies, including:

Alpha herpesviruses are the causative agents of acute infections and are generally linked to sores or ulcerations that appear on the skin or mucous membranes. Herpes simplex virus type 1 and varicella-zoster virus are both types of alpha herpesviruses. Both of these viruses can cause genital herpes.
Beta herpesviruses are a group of viruses that are known to produce dormant infections and are often linked to the development of chronic illnesses. Examples of beta herpesviruses include the cytomegalovirus and the human herpesvirus 6.

In most cases, cancers and lymphoproliferative diseases are connected with gamma herpesviruses because these viruses generate latent infections. The Epstein-Barr virus and the Kaposi's sarcoma-associated herpesvirus are both examples of gamma herpesviruses.

DNA viruses are known as papillomaviruses, and they are responsible for a wide range of diseases, including warts and some forms of cancer. The genomes of papillomaviruses are composed of double-stranded DNA, and the replication process is catalyzed by a viral DNA-dependent DNA polymerase.

In accordance with the genetic and antigenic properties that they share, papillomaviruses can be further subdivided into a number of different genera. Many different diseases can be brought on by a single genus, and certain genera have been linked to an increased likelihood of cancer.

RNA viruses known as orthomyxoviruses are responsible for a wide range of infections, including the influenza virus. The genomes of orthomyxoviruses are composed of antisense RNA, and the replication process is catalyzed by an RNA-dependent RNA polymerase produced by the virus. Orthomyxoviruses can be further classified into several genera, including:

This virus is capable of infecting a wide range of hosts, including human beings, pigs, and birds. Influenza A virus is associated with seasonal flu outbreaks and pandemics.

Although it is capable of infecting humans, this virus does not typically cause widespread outbreaks. In most cases, epidemics of seasonal influenza are caused by the Influenza B virus.

This virus is capable of infecting humans, however it is not as widespread and does not cause as much illness as influenza A or B viruses.

The replication process of viruses is unique in that it requires the help of a host cell. After it has successfully entered the cell of its host, the virus will use the machinery of the host cell to copy its genetic material and make new viral particles. This process has the potential to damage the host cell, which may ultimately result in an ailment or disease.

The capacity of viruses for rapid evolution is also a crucial aspect in the manner in which they function. Viruses are capable of undergoing mutations, which can either enable them to evade the immune system of their host or make them more contagious. Because of this, it may be difficult to create therapies that are successful as well as immunizations.

One of the most significant factors in how viruses work is their ability to spread from person to person. There are several different ways in which viruses can spread, including the following:

When virus particles are dispersed through the air, which typically happens when someone coughs or sneezes, this is known as airborne transmission. The influenza virus and the measles virus are both examples of viruses that are capable of spreading through airborne transmission.

When someone comes into direct contact with a person who is infected with a virus, or when they come into contact with a surface that is contaminated with viruses, this is known as contact transmission. The virus that causes the common cold and the norovirus are both examples of viruses that can be passed from person to person by direct contact.

The transmission of a virus through the bite of an infected animal or insect is referred to as vector-borne transmission. The Zika virus and the West Nile virus are both examples of viruses that can be transmitted via vectors.

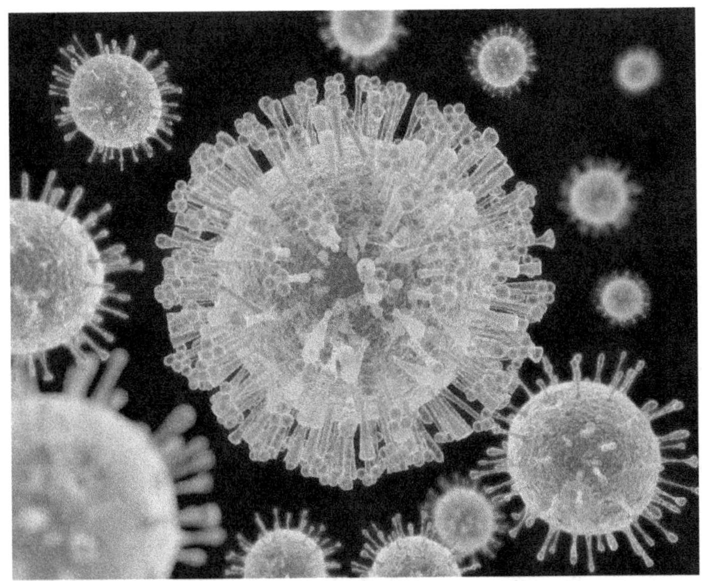

It is vital to both prevent and cure viral infections if one wishes to reduce the negative effects that viral risks have on public health. The following are some of the most effective prevention and treatment strategies for viral infections:

Vaccinations are among the most successful means of warding off diseases caused by viruses. Vaccines operate by inducing the immune system to develop antibodies against the virus, which either stops an illness from occurring or lessens the severity of the symptoms that an infection causes.

Antiviral medications can be used to treat viral infections. These drugs are effective because they target particular stages of the life cycle of the virus, thereby preventing the virus from replicating and spreading.

In order to prevent the spread of viral diseases, it is possible to use public health measures such as testing, the tracking of contacts, and quarantine. Outbreaks of viruses such as Ebola and SARS have been successfully contained as a result of these preventative efforts.

It is possible to lessen the spread of infectious diseases by taking preventative steps on an individual level, such as washing one's hands often, wearing masks, and maintaining social distance. The transmission of respiratory viruses like influenza and COVID-19 has been significantly slowed as a direct result of the implementation of these preventative measures.

In conclusion, viruses are one of the most significant threats facing public health today. When it comes to preventing and treating viral infections, having a solid understanding of the structure and behavior of viruses is absolutely necessary. Viruses are special in that they have the potential to swiftly adapt and transmit from one person to another. This makes it difficult to keep viruses under control.

Vaccination, antiviral medication, public health measures, and personal protective measures are just some of the many methods that can be utilized in conjunction with one another to effectively prevent and cure viral infections. It is absolutely necessary to carry on research and make investments in public health infrastructure and pandemic preparedness in order to reduce the negative effects of any future virus dangers.

We can lessen the impact that viral dangers have on public health, the economy of the world, and everyday life if we maintain our level of investment in efforts to prevent and treat infectious diseases.

Overview of the immune system and how it works to protect against viruses

The immune system is a complex network of cells, tissues, and organs that work together to protect the body from infectious agents like viruses. This network is known as the immune system. The immune system is essential in preventing viral infections, and understanding its function is critical in developing effective treatments and vaccines.

Its primary function is to prevent illness. Understanding the components of the immune system is vital to the creation of successful therapies and vaccinations because it is the immune system that is responsible for preventing and controlling illnesses. In this section, we will present an overview of the many components of the immune system. These components include the innate immune system, the adaptive immune system, and the lymphatic system.

When it comes to fighting against infectious invaders, the innate immune system is the first line of protection. It is made up of cells and tissues that are able to identify and react to a wide variety of infectious agents, such as viruses, bacteria, and fungus.

The cells that are part of the body's first line of defense include:
Neutrophils are the most common type of white blood cell found in the body, and they are also the first sort of white blood cell to react to an infection after it has taken hold. They are phagocytic cells that can engulf and destroy pathogens. The production of neutrophils can speedily increase in response to bacterial infections, which is

important because they are necessary for the prevention and management of bacterial infections.

Macrophages are another type of phagocytic cell that has the ability to consume and eliminate harmful microorganisms. They are found in all of the tissues of the body and play a crucial part in the process that sets off the immune response. Macrophages have the ability to identify and react to a wide variety of infections. In addition, macrophages are capable of producing cytokines, which can stimulate the activity of other immune system cells.

Natural killer cells have the ability to identify and eliminate cancer cells as well as cells infected with viruses. They have a significant role in the suppression of viral infections and the prevention of the formation of tumors. Natural killer cells have the ability to create cytokines, which have the potential to activate other cells within the immune system, such as macrophages and dendritic cells.

Dendritic cells can be found in tissues that are constantly exposed to the outside world, such as the skin and the mucosal surfaces of the body. They can recognize and capture pathogens and present them to other cells of the immune system to initiate an immune response. The stimulation of dendritic cells can lead to the activation and multiplication of B cells and T cells, which are both crucial steps in the process of initiating the adaptive immune response. Dendritic cells are a key component of this process.

Mast cells are tissue-resident cells that, in response to infections or other stimuli, are able to create the inflammatory mediators histamine and other mediators of inflammation. Innate immune responses, such as those to parasites and other pathogens, are orchestrated in large part by mast cells, which play an important part in these processes.

Eosinophils are a particular kind of white blood cell that play an important role in the body's immune response to parasites and other infectious agents. They are capable of producing cytokines, which can activate other cells of the immune system, and they are also capable of releasing toxic granules, which are capable of killing infections. White blood cells known as basophils play an important role in the immune system's fight against parasites and other infectious agents. They can produce histamine and other mediators of inflammation in response to pathogens or other stimuli and play a critical role in the innate immune response.
Additionally, the innate immune system is comprised of a variety of proteins and chemicals that are able to identify pathogens and react appropriately to them. These include the following:
The complement system is made up of many proteins that have the ability to identify and eliminate harmful organisms. The complement system can be triggered by antibodies or directly by pathogens. Once activated, the complement system can lead to the killing of pathogens by a variety of methods, including as the development of pores in the pathogen's membrane and the activation of phagocytic cells. Antibodies and pathogens both have the ability to activate the complement system.

Cytokines are tiny proteins that can influence the immune response by boosting inflammation, activating immune cells, and causing cell death in infected cells. Cytokines are secreted by activated immune cells in response to infections. Cytokines can be produced by a variety of immune system cells, including macrophages, dendritic cells, and T cells; the production of these cytokines can be stimulated by the presence of pathogens or other stimuli. Cytokines play an important role in the immunological response.

Proteins known as interferons are capable of inhibiting the multiplication of viruses and stimulating the immune system. Interferons are produced by virus-infected cells and can stimulate nearby cells to produce antiviral proteins that can prevent viral replication. Natural killer cells and T cells, both of which have the ability to identify and eliminate virus-infected cells, can be activated by interferons.

The adaptive immune system is made up of cells and tissues that are able to recognize and react to a variety of different viruses and other types of infectious agents. The adaptive immune system, in contrast to the innate immune system, which provides a general protection against a wide range of diseases, is able to provide a specific defense against a particular pathogen. The cells of the adaptive immune system include:

B cells have the ability to create antibodies, which are proteins that are able to identify and inhibit the activity of viruses. B cells have the ability to recognize and react to a wide range of viral antigens, and the activation of these cells can result in the generation of vast quantities of particular antibodies that are able to bind to and inhibit the activity of viruses.

T cells can recognize and kill virus-infected cells directly and can also help activate other cells of the immune system. T cells are able to recognize viral antigens when they are presented to them by infected cells; this recognition can then lead to the activation of T cells, which in turn can lead to the destruction of infected cells and the removal of the virus.

Additionally, the adaptive immune system is comprised of a wide variety of chemicals and proteins that are able to recognize specific diseases and react appropriately to them. These include the following:

Antibodies are proteins that are produced by B cells, and they are able to identify and inhibit the activity of viruses. Antibodies have the ability to bind to viral antigens and so block the viral antigens' ability to enter cells or interact with cellular receptors. Antibodies have the ability to stimulate other cells of the immune system, such as macrophages and natural killer cells, to engage in the process of destroying virus-infected cells after they have been activated.

MHC molecules are molecules that stimulate an immune response by presenting viral antigens to T lymphocytes. Infected cells have MHC molecules on their surface, and these molecules have the ability to deliver viral antigens that are made by the virus inside the infected cell. The presentation of viral antigens by MHC molecules can lead to the activation of T cells, which can recognize and kill infected cells.

On the surface of T cells contain molecules called T cell receptors, which are able to identify viral antigens when they are presented by MHC molecules. T cell receptors are able to recognize a specific viral antigen due to their high level of specificity. The activation of T lymphocytes by viral antigens can result in the death of infected cells and the complete removal of the virus from the body.

The lymphatic system is a network of tubes and tissues that plays an important role in the movement of immune cells and fluids throughout the body. Lymph nodes, the spleen, the thymus, and bone marrow are all components of the lymphatic system. These organs all play a role in the generation of immune cells, as well as their maturation and activation.

Lymph nodes are bean-shaped structures that are dispersed throughout the body and play a role in the activation of immune cells. Lymph nodes can be identified by their characteristic small size. Lymph nodes contain B cells, T cells, and dendritic cells, and their activation can lead to the generation of antibodies that are specific as well as the activation of T cells that are specific.

The spleen is an organ that may be found in the upper left side of the abdomen. It plays a role in the process of activating and destroying immune cells. Activation of the spleen's B cells, T cells, macrophages, and dendritic cells can result in the creation of particular antibodies and the death of infected cells in the body.

The maturation of T cells requires the participation of a gland called the thymus, which is found in the chest. The thymus contains specialized cells that are able to stimulate the maturation of T lymphocytes and their activation in response to viral antigens. This might help stop the virus from spreading further.

The bone marrow is a type of tissue that can be found inside of bones and plays an important role in the generation of immune cells. These cells include B cells, T cells, and natural killer cells. The bone marrow contains specialized cells that can promote the production and maturation of immune cells, and its activation can lead to the production of specific antibodies and the activation of specific T cells.

How viruses affect the body and how the immune system responds

A vast variety of diseases in humans, animals, and plants can be brought on by viruses, which are little infectious organisms. Viruses are exceptional in that they can only replicate inside host cells, escape the immune system, and result in long-lasting infections. In this section, we'll talk about how viruses affect the human body and how the immune system responds to viral infections.

Virus type and the host's immunological response can have a big impact on how viruses affect the body. While some viruses only cause minor symptoms, others can lead to life-threatening disease or even death. The incubation period, prodromal period, and acute phase are the three stages of a viral infection's consequences. The incubation period is a crucial period in the development of infectious diseases. The infection is growing in the body throughout this time, although the person is typically asymptomatic. Depending on the pathogen, the incubation period might last anything from a few hours to several weeks.

Infectious disease transmission depends on the incubation period. The individual may be asymptomatic but continue spreading the infection and potentially infecting others throughout this time. This is especially important for respiratory infections like COVID-19 because people can spread the infection even before showing symptoms. The following variables can affect how long the incubation phase lasts:

Different pathogens have different incubation periods. In the case of influenza, the incubation period normally lasts between one and four days, whereas the incubation period for hepatitis B can last for as long as six months.

The duration of the incubation period is susceptible to being influenced by the virulence of the infection. More virulent pathogens can cause symptoms more quickly than less virulent pathogens.

There is a correlation between the quantity of the pathogen and the duration of the incubation period. It may take a longer time for a lower dose of the pathogen to produce symptoms compared to a greater dose.

The incubation period might be lengthened or shortened, depending on the individual's immune system. A prolonged duration of incubation may be the result of a stronger immune system that is able to keep the virus at bay for a longer amount of time.

The length of time an infectious disease spends "incubating" is a crucial factor in both the diagnosis and treatment of infectious diseases. When medical practitioners have a thorough understanding of the incubation period, they are better able to pinpoint the infectious agent that is responsible for the sickness and establish effective treatment plans.

For instance, if an individual shows symptoms of a respiratory infection but the incubation period for COVID-19 is two weeks, the healthcare professional may need to examine other potential infections and run more tests to confirm the diagnosis.

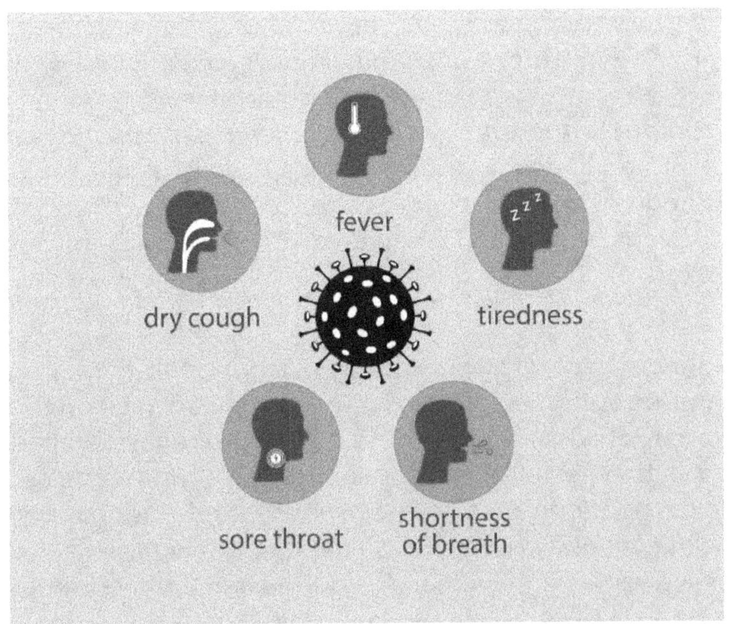

In the treatment of infectious disorders, the duration of the incubation period is also a significant consideration. When a patient is diagnosed and given treatment at an earlier stage, their chances of recovery and the lower risk they pose to others. On the other hand, early diagnosis can be difficult to achieve due to the fact that the individual will normally exhibit no symptoms during the incubation period.

During an infectious disease, the time that passes before the beginning of symptoms and after the sickness reaches its worst is referred to as the prodromal period. This stage is significant in the progression of the disease since it marks the slow development of symptoms and is defined by the gradual development of symptoms. In this section, we will talk about the prodromal phase, why it is so important to the progression of disease, and how it plays a part in the diagnosis and treatment of infectious diseases.

The prodromal period is the period of time between the start of symptoms and the illness's peak. During this time, the affected individual could feel a variety of symptoms, such as weariness, fever, headache, and aches and pains in their muscles. It is possible for the duration of the prodromal stage to change based on the infectious agent as well as the individual's immune system.

The prodromal period is an important phase in the progression of infectious diseases. During this time, the immune system is preparing to launch an attack on the virus, while at the same time, the pathogen is quickly replicating itself. The severity of the prodromal stage as well as how long it lasts can provide valuable insight about the infectious agent as well as the immunological response of the individual. The duration of the prodromal stage, as well as its severity, can be influenced by a number of factors, including the following:
Different pathogens can cause different prodromal periods. For instance, the prodromal phase of influenza can last anywhere from one to four days, but the prodromal phase of hepatitis B might last anywhere from one week to several weeks.

It is possible for the virulence of the virus to have an impact on how severe the prodromal stage is. During the prodromal period, symptoms that are more severe can be caused by infections that are more virulent.
The individual's immune system can have an effect on the intensity of the symptoms as well as the amount of time they continue during the prodromal period. There is a correlation between having a stronger immune system and being able to confine the virus more rapidly, which can lead to a shorter prodromal period.

The prodromal period is important in the diagnosis and treatment of infectious diseases. The severity of the prodromal stage as well as how long it lasts can provide valuable insight about the infectious agent as well as the immunological response of the individual. This information can assist medical experts in determining the specific pathogen that is responsible for generating the sickness and in designing effective treatment options.

For instance, if an individual goes through a prodromal stage that lasts for a significant amount of time, the healthcare professional may need to investigate a pathogen that causes chronic infections, such as HIV or hepatitis B. If an individual has a brief prodromal phase yet gets significant symptoms during the acute phase, the healthcare practitioner may need to investigate a more virulent pathogen as the likely cause of the illness.
The prodromal phase is also an essential part of the therapy process for infectious disorders. The earlier a patient is diagnosed and treated, the better their chances of recovery and the lower risk they pose to others. Early identification can be difficult, though, because the prodromal period isn't always consistent or clear-cut like other stages of the disease.

The acute phase is the period of an infectious disease during which the pathogen is actively replicating in the body and the individual is experiencing symptoms. This phase often comes after the prodromal period, which is the time when the individual may have had non-specific symptoms like as weariness, fever, and aches and pains in their muscles.

During the acute phase, the immune system is aggressively responding to the pathogen in an effort to eradicate it from the body. During this phase, the condition is known as an acute infection. The development of symptoms including fever, inflammation, and damage to tissue may be a consequence of this immunological response.

It is possible for the severity and duration of the acute phase to change depending on the pathogen as well as the immune system of the individual. The acute phase may be modest and pass quickly in some situations, while in other cases it may be severe and linger for a number of weeks or months. This can depend on the individual case. The severity and length of the acute phase can be influenced by a number of factors, including the following: The acute phase can have varying degrees of severity and last for varying amounts of time depending on the pathogen that caused it. For example, influenza typically causes a short and severe acute phase, while HIV can cause a prolonged and variable acute phase.

It is possible for the virulence of the pathogen to influence how severe the acute phase is. Symptoms that are more severe and that last for a longer period of time during the acute phase can be caused by more virulent microorganisms.

The degree of severity and length of time spent in the acute phase are both influenced by the individual's immune system. A more robust immune system may be better able to eradicate the pathogen in a shorter amount of time, which would result in a more manageable length of time spent in the acute phase.
When it comes to the diagnosis and treatment of infectious diseases, the acute phase is extremely crucial. The intensity of the acute phase, as well as how long it lasts, can provide valuable insight into the infectious

agent as well as the individual's immunological response. This information can assist medical experts in determining the specific pathogen that is responsible for generating the sickness and in designing effective treatment options.

For instance, if a person goes through a severe acute phase, the healthcare professional may need to evaluate the possibility of a more virulent disease or a weakened immune system. If an individual experiences a prolonged acute phase, the healthcare professional may need to consider a pathogen that causes chronic infections, such as HIV or hepatitis B.

The treatment of infectious diseases also places a significant emphasis on the acute phase. The earlier a patient is diagnosed and treated, the better their chances of recovery and the lower risk they pose to others. During the acute phase of the disease, therapeutic techniques may concentrate on symptom management and bolstering the immunological response. Antiviral drugs may, in certain circumstances, be utilized in order to directly target the infection.

It is possible for a viral infection to have quite different effects on the body depending not just on the type of virus but also on the immunological response of the host. While some viruses may only cause moderate symptoms, others have the potential to cause severe disease or even death.
When it comes to protecting the body from viral infections, the immune system is an extremely important player. The immune system can recognize and respond to viral infections by activating immune cells and producing antibodies and cytokines that can inhibit viral replication and eliminate infected cells. Both the innate immune

response and the adaptive immune response can be broken down into two distinct phases when discussing the immune system's reaction to viral infections.

The initial line of protection that the body has against foreign invaders is called the innate immune response. It is a non-specific reaction that is present from birth and does not require previous exposure to a specific pathogen. In other words, it is an innate immune response. The innate immune response is made up of a few different parts, the most notable of which are the physical and chemical barriers, the cells, and the soluble proteins. These parts cooperate with one another to identify and eradicate diseases that have gained access to the body.

Physical barriers are the pathogens' first line of defense against the host. They consist of the mucous membranes, which line the respiratory, gastrointestinal, and urogenital tracts and trap pathogens; the skin, which acts as a physical barrier to prevent pathogens from entering the body; and the mucus membranes of the mouth and nose, which also serve the same purpose.

Chemical barriers are also important in the innate immune response. They include enzymes such as lysozyme, which break down the cell walls of bacteria, and acidic environments, such as in the stomach, which can kill pathogens.

The innate immune response involves participation from a variety of cell types, including the following: Phagocytes, which include macrophages and neutrophils, are specialized immune system cells that have the ability to consume and destroy harmful microorganisms. NK cells are a specific type of white blood cell that have the ability to identify and eliminate abnormal or infectious cells found in the body.

Dendritic cells are specialized immune system cells that have the ability to communicate foreign antigens to other cells of the immune system, thereby stimulating an immunological response.
There is also a significant role for soluble proteins in the innate immune response. Some examples of these proteins include complement proteins and cytokines. Complement proteins can coat pathogens, making them more susceptible to elimination by phagocytes. Cytokines, on the other hand, can promote inflammation and recruit immune cells to the site of an infection. Both of these processes are necessary for an effective immune response.

When it comes to defending the body against infectious diseases, the innate immune response is one of the most important factors. It provides immediate protection against a range of pathogens, including those that have not been encountered before.

However, there are circumstances in which the innate immune response may not be adequate to eliminate the pathogen, and in these situations, an adaptive immune response may be necessary. The adaptive immune response is a highly targeted response that has to have previous experience with a particular pathogen in order to develop.

The adaptive immune response is a type of immune response that develops after initial exposure to a pathogen but only in response to that particular pathogen. The stimulation of immune cells and the creation of particular antibodies are both necessary steps in this complex procedure. The humoral immune response and the cell-mediated immune response are the two primary components that make up the adaptive immune response.

The process of producing antibodies in response to a particular disease is known as humoral immunity and it is carried out by B cells. B cells are a type of white blood cell that have the ability to identify particular antigens that are found on the surface of a disease. Once activated, B cells can differentiate into plasma cells, which produce large amounts of antibodies that can bind to the pathogen and neutralize it.

The activation of T cells in response to a particular pathogen is the first step in the process of cell-mediated immunity. T cells are a type of white blood cell that have the ability to detect particular antigens that are found on the surface of a disease. T cells are capable of differentiating into a variety of cell types once they have been activated. These cell types include cytotoxic T cells, which are able to directly destroy infected cells, and helper T cells, which are able to stimulate other immune cells.

Antigen-presenting cells, which include dendritic cells and macrophages, are essential to the adaptive immune response and play an important part in the process. These cells have the ability to ingest and process infections, after which they can convey bits of the pathogen's antigens to other immune cells in order to initiate an immune response.

When a pathogen goes into the body and is recognized by immune cells, this triggers the adaptive immune response. Adaptive immunity is a more sophisticated kind of immunity. The pathogen's antigens are presented to B cells and T cells, activating them and initiating the production of antibodies and the activation of other immune cells.

Memory cells can be generated by the adaptive immune response after an individual has been exposed to a particular pathogen. These memory cells are able to detect the pathogen and respond to it in a more prompt and effective manner upon subsequent exposure. This memory reaction is the foundation of vaccination, which entails exposing the body to a form of a pathogen that has been weakened or rendered inactive in order to establish a memory response without actually causing disease.

The adaptive immune response is an extremely important component in the whole process of defending the body against infectious illnesses. It is able to zero in on and eliminate specific pathogens, as well as develop memory cells that can offer long-term protection against recurrent infections.

However, there are circumstances in which the adaptive immune response might not be adequate to eradicate the virus. In these scenarios, it might be necessary to resort to additional treatments, such as antiviral drugs or immunomodulatory therapy.

Viruses have developed a wide variety of evasion mechanisms over the course of evolution, which allow them to establish persistent infections. Some of these strategies include:

Certain viruses are capable of altering the antigens on their surface in order to avoid being recognized by the immune system. Some viruses are able to form latent infections in the cells of their hosts, which allows them to avoid being detected by the immune system because they are not actively multiplying.

Some viruses are able to inhibit the immunological response of the host, which enables the virus to reproduce and spread disease without being destroyed by the body's defenses. There are viruses that can cause immunological tolerance, which is when the immune system is unable to effectively generate a response against the virus.

Because of these techniques, viruses are able to form chronic infections, a condition in which the virus remains dormant in the body for extended periods of time and is able to inflict ongoing damage to the tissues and organs of the host.

In summary, viruses are responsible for a diverse array of diseases that can affect humans, animals, and plants. It is possible for a viral infection to have quite different effects on the body depending not just on the type of virus but also on the immunological response of the host. While some viruses may only cause moderate symptoms, others have the potential to cause severe disease or even death.

When it comes to protecting the body from viral infections, the immune system is an extremely important player. The innate immune response offers protection against a wide variety of pathogens, but the adaptive immune response offers protection against a specific pathogen and has the potential to offer long-term immunity against subsequent infections.

There are a variety of methods that viruses have developed to escape detection by the immune system and to create persistent infections. In order to create successful therapies and vaccines for viral infections, it is essential to have a solid understanding of these techniques. Our understanding of viral pathogenesis and the creation of efficient treatments and vaccines will both benefit from the continuation of research into the effects of viruses on the body and the immune response to viral infections.

CHAPTER II

Herbal Antivirals: An Overview

Explanation of what herbal antivirals are and how they work

Herbal antivirals are natural substances that are produced from plants and have been found to have antiviral activities. These substances have been called phytochemicals. They have a long history of application in the treatment and prevention of viral infections in conventional medical practice. In this section, we will explain what herbal antivirals are, how they combat viral infections, and the possible benefits of using herbal antivirals to both prevent and treat viral illnesses.

Herbal antivirals are organic compounds made from plants that have been demonstrated to have antiviral effects. They are frequently used in conjunction with other treatments, such as antiviral drugs, as they are effective in both the prevention and treatment of viral infections. Numerous medicinal plants, including herbs, have been identified as having antiviral effects. Some of the most commonly used herbal antivirals include: Echinacea is a well-known herb that has a long history of use as an immune system booster as well as a means of both preventing and treating viral illnesses, such as the common cold and the flu. It has been demonstrated that garlic is a powerful herb that possesses antiviral capabilities. It has the potential to strengthen one's immune system and protect against viral illnesses like the common cold and the flu.

Elderberry is a natural antiviral that has been shown to be effective against a range of viruses, including influenza and herpes simplex virus. In conventional medicine, licorice root is a well-known herb that has been utilized for the treatment of viral infections for many decades. It has been demonstrated that it is effective against viruses and that it can help strengthen the immune system. It has been demonstrated that ginger, a naturally occurring antiviral, is effective against a variety of viruses, including influenza and respiratory syncytial virus (RSV).

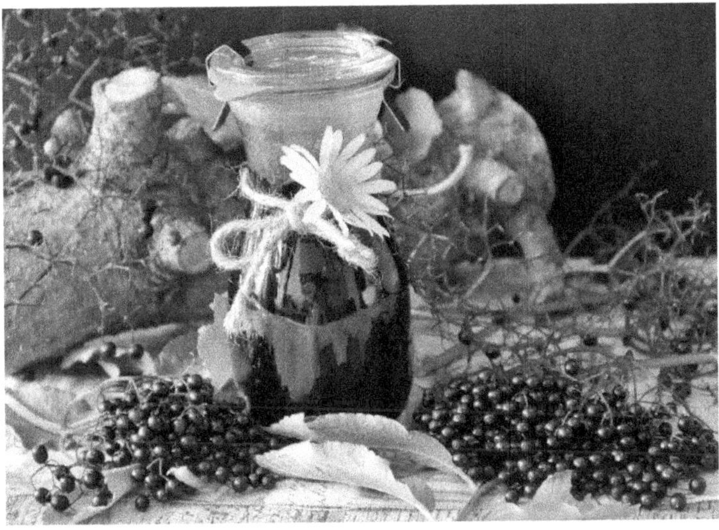

Herbal antivirals activate the immune system while also inhibiting virus multiplication. They accomplish this through a variety of different ways. Some of the most common mechanisms of action include:

Numerous antiviral herbs include specific compounds that research has shown to be effective at preventing the replication of viruses. These substances may prevent the virus from attaching to host cells, penetrating the cell membrane, or replicating within the host cell by interfering with its ability to do these things. For example, some herbs contain compounds that can inhibit the activity of the viral polymerase enzyme, which is required for viral replication.

It is possible for certain herbal antivirals to stimulate the immune system, thereby increasing the body's capacity to ward off diseases. Herbs such as echinacea and astragalus, for instance, have the potential to boost the function of natural killer cells and increase the creation of cytokines, which are critical components of the immune system's communication molecules.

Some herbal antivirals can directly kill viruses. It has been demonstrated that tea tree oil possesses direct virucidal effect against a variety of viruses, including the herpes simplex virus and the influenza virus, among others. When it comes to the prevention and treatment of viral infections, the use of herbal antivirals presents a number of possible benefits that patients can take advantage of. Some of these benefits include:

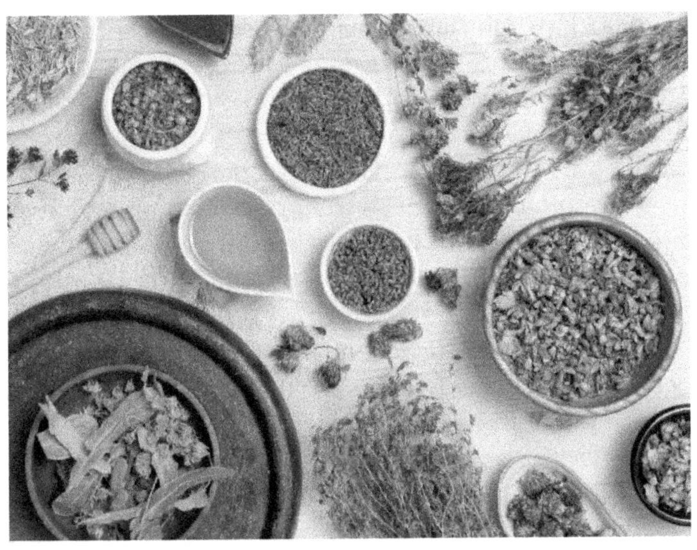

Herbal antivirals are natural chemicals obtained from plants and are, in most cases, not thought to pose any health risks. In comparison to traditional pharmaceuticals, which frequently come with a number of negative side effects, these have a decreased potential for adverse reactions.

Echinacea and garlic are just two examples of the many natural antivirals that can help strengthen the immune system and improve its capacity to ward off infections.

Many herbal antivirals contain specific compounds that have been shown to have antiviral activity against specific viruses. Conventional drugs, which may have a wider range of activity, may not be as successful in treating viral infections as this tailored activity, which can be more effective in treating viral infections.

When compared to traditional antiviral drugs, herbal antivirals typically have lower price tags, which makes them a more cost-effective choice for both preventing and treating viral infections.

In conclusion, herbal antivirals are natural chemicals derived from plants that have been found to have antiviral effects. These substances have been shown to inhibit the growth of some viruses. They are frequently used in conjunction with other treatments, such as antiviral drugs, as they are effective in both the prevention and treatment of viral infections. Herbal antivirals fight viral infections in a number of different methods, including bolstering the immune system and interfering with the multiplication of viruses. They can be used both to prevent and treat viral infections. They have the potential to provide a number of benefits, including as a lower risk of adverse effects, improved immune system function, cost-effective antiviral action, and tailored antiviral activity. However, it is important to note that herbal antivirals are not a replacement for medical care, and patients should always discuss their use with a member of their healthcare team prior to utilizing any herbal remedies.

Ongoing research is being conducted to investigate the efficacy and safety of herbal antivirals, and this research will help us gain a better knowledge of the possible benefits and limitations of herbal antivirals. The use of herbal antivirals should be examined in the context of an individual's general health and medical history. Herbal antivirals offer a promising alternative or supplementary therapy in the prevention and treatment of viral infections.

Overview of the different types of herbal antivirals

Herbal antivirals are natural substances that are produced from plants and have been found to have antiviral activities. They have a long history of application in the treatment and prevention of viral infections in conventional medical practice. In this section, we will go over a general overview of the many types of herbal antivirals, including their characteristics, applications, and possible advantages.

Echinacea is a herb used for ages in conventional medicine to strengthen the immune system and cure a range of ailments, including viral infections. In recent years, it has become increasingly popular as a natural therapy for the treatment and prevention of the flu and the common cold.
Echinacea is known to contain a number of different compounds, some of which have been found to have immunomodulatory and antiviral effects. These chemicals include polysaccharides, glycoproteins, and alkamides. It has been demonstrated that it increases the synthesis of cytokines, which are vital immune response mediators, as well as stimulates the activity of immune cells such natural killer cells, macrophages, and T-cells. Additionally, echinacea contains a number of antioxidants, which work to shield the body from the damaging effects of oxidative stress and inflammation.

Echinacea has a long history of usage as a remedy for a variety of illnesses and conditions, including the prevention and treatment of viral infections like the common cold and influenza. It has also been used to treat other respiratory infections, such as bronchitis and sinusitis, as well as urinary tract infections and skin infections. Echinacea can be purchased in a number of different preparations, including as capsules, pills, tinctures, and teas.

It has been demonstrated that echinacea increases the production of cytokines, which are significant immune response mediators, as well as the activity of immune cells such as macrophages, natural killer cells, and T- cells. Additionally, echinacea has been proven to boost the activity of immune cells such as natural killer cells and T-cells. This contributes to the enhancement of the body's natural defenses against viral infections and other pathogens in the environment.

Echinacea has been demonstrated to be useful in lowering the severity of symptoms and length of time spent suffering from the flu and the common cold. Echinacea, according to the findings of a number of different studies, can help to alleviate symptoms like coughing, congestion, and sore throats, and it also has the potential to help prevent recurring infections.

Echinacea is known to include a number of antioxidants, which work to shield the body from the damaging effects of free radicals and inflammation. This may aid in the reduction of inflammation throughout the body and aid in the prevention of chronic diseases such as cancer and heart disease.

It has been demonstrated that echinacea speeds up the healing process of wounds and lowers the likelihood of infection. It is possible that its ability to boost the immune system and reduce inflammation, along with its antibacterial and antiviral capabilities, are responsible for this effect.

Echinacea has been shown to be effective in treating a number of skin issues, such as eczema, psoriasis, and acne. Because of its anti-inflammatory and antibacterial qualities, it could be able to help reduce inflammation and stop the growth of germs, both of which are factors that might contribute to these illnesses.

Although echinacea is thought to be safe for the vast majority of people, it has been linked to a number of adverse events in a some individuals, including allergic reactions, gastrointestinal distress, and headaches. It is also possible for it to interact negatively with other medications, particularly immunosuppressants and certain chemotherapy treatments. Before using Echinacea, it is essential to discuss the supplement with a qualified medical professional, particularly if you are pregnant or breastfeeding, or if you are currently taking any medications.

Due of the beneficial effects it has on health, garlic has been cultivated and used since ancient times. It belongs to the Allium family, which also contains shallots, onions, and leeks. Allicin, sulfur compounds, and flavonoids are only some of the components that are found in high concentrations in garlic. These compounds have been demonstrated to have a variety of positive effects on human health.

The therapeutic qualities of garlic are due to the presence of a number of compounds that are only found in garlic. Garlic gets its intense smell from a molecule called allicin, which is also one of the most important active compounds in garlic. It has been established that it is effective against bacterial infections, viral infections, and fungal infections. Garlic contains a variety of sulfur compounds, including diallyl disulfide and S-allyl cysteine, which all work together to give it its therapeutic qualities. Antioxidants like flavonoids, which include quercetin and kaempferol, assist the body in defending itself against the damaging effects of oxidative stress and inflammation.

Garlic has a long history of use for its purported medical benefits, and recent scientific investigation has borne out many of the functions traditionally attributed to it. It is available in several forms, including fresh garlic, garlic supplements, and garlic oil.

It has been demonstrated that garlic has the ability to enhance the activity of immune cells such as macrophages and natural killer cells. These cells play an important role in defending the body against viral infections and other pathogens.

Individuals who suffer from hypertension may benefit from garlic's ability to bring their blood pressure down. According to the findings of a number of different research, taking garlic supplements can dramatically lower both the systolic and diastolic blood pressure.

Research has revealed that eating garlic can help lower cholesterol levels in individuals who already have high levels. Garlic supplements have been shown in a number of trials to bring about reductions in total cholesterol, LDL cholesterol, and triglyceride levels.

It has been demonstrated that garlic has various benefits for the health of the cardiovascular system. It has the potential to lower blood pressure, cholesterol levels, and prevent the formation of blood clots, all of which are risk factors for cardiovascular diseases such as heart attacks and strokes.

It has been demonstrated that garlic contains anticancer qualities, and these properties may aid in preventing the development of several different types of cancer, including colorectal, breast, and prostate cancer.

Garlic has been traditionally used to treat respiratory infections, such as the common cold and flu. It has been demonstrated to possess antiviral characteristics, which suggests that it may assist to lessen the severity of these diseases and shorten their duration.

A variety of skin illnesses, including acne and athlete's foot, have been successfully treated with garlic in the past. Because of its antibacterial and antifungal qualities, it may help to inhibit the growth of bacteria and fungi, both of which are known to be associated with these disorders.

It has been shown that garlic speeds up the healing process for wounds and may also aid to prevent infections. Its antibacterial characteristics may assist to lower the risk of infection, and its anti-inflammatory properties may help to reduce inflammation and improve healing. The combination of these two types of features may help to minimize the likelihood of infection.

Research has shown that garlic has a number of positive effects on the digestive system. It has the potential to assist in the reduction of inflammation in the digestive tract, the enhancement of digestion, and the prevention of the growth of bacteria that are pathogenic in the gut.

Garlic has been shown to enhance athletic performance and may help to reduce fatigue and improve endurance. It is possible that the antioxidant capabilities of this substance will assist in lowering the levels of oxidative stress and inflammation in the body, both of which can contribute to weariness and injury to the muscles.

Garlic is thought to be perfectly safe for the vast majority of people, although it is possible for some individuals to experience adverse reactions to it, such as gastrointestinal distress and allergic reactions. It is also possible for it to interact negatively with other drugs, such as those used to thin the blood or treat HIV. Garlic should not be used without first discussing its use with a qualified medical professional, particularly if you are pregnant or breastfeeding or if you are currently taking any drugs.

Elderberry is a plant that has been utilized for the treatment of a variety of medical conditions for ages. Although it was originally from Europe, it has subsequently become naturalized in a great many other regions of the world, including North America. Elderberry is loaded with a number of different chemicals, such as anthocyanins, flavonoids, and phenolic acids, all of which have been demonstrated to have a variety of positive effects on human health.

Elderberry is known to have therapeutic value due to the presence of a number of different chemicals within the fruit. Elderberries are a type of flavonoid that are known for their distinctive dark purple hue, which is caused by anthocyanins. They are known as antioxidants, and they aid in the protection of the body against oxidative stress as well as inflammation. Elderberry also contains flavonoids, the likes of which have been demonstrated to possess antiviral, anti-inflammatory, and antioxidant properties. Examples of these flavonoids are quercetin and kaempferol. Phenolic acids, such as caffeic acid and chlorogenic acid, are also present in elderberry and have been shown to have anti-inflammatory and antioxidant properties.

Elderberry has a long history of use for its claimed medical benefits, and recent scientific investigation has backed up a good number of those traditional applications. It can be obtained in a variety of formats, including as dietary supplements, beverages (such tea or supplements), and syrup made from elderberries.

The activity of immune cells, such as natural killer cells, which aid in protecting the body against viral infections and other pathogens can be boosted by elderberry, according to a number of scientific studies.

Elderberry has a long history of usage in traditional medicine for the treatment of cold and flu symptoms, and multiple studies have demonstrated that it is helpful in doing so. It has been shown to lessen the intensity of cold and flu symptoms, including fever, cough, and congestion, as well as shorten their duration.

Studies have indicated that individuals who already have high cholesterol can benefit from elderberry's ability to reduce their cholesterol levels. According to the findings of a number of different research, taking elderberry supplements can bring total cholesterol and LDL cholesterol levels down.

It has been established that elderberry provides a number of benefits for the health of the heart. It can help to lower blood pressure, reduce inflammation, and improve circulation, which can help to reduce the risk of cardiovascular disease.

It has been established that elderberry provides a number of benefits for the health of the skin. It can help to reduce inflammation, increase skin hydration, and protect against oxidative stress, all of which are factors that can contribute to the formation of wrinkles and other symptoms of aging in the skin.

Elderberry has been identified as possessing anticancer qualities and has the potential to aid in the prevention of the development of a variety of cancers, including breast, colon, and prostate cancer.

It has been demonstrated that elderberry has a number of positive effects on the digestive system. It has the potential to assist in the reduction of inflammation in the digestive tract, the enhancement of digestion, and the prevention of the growth of bacteria that are pathogenic in the gut.

It has been demonstrated that elderberry has a number of positive effects on cognitive performance. Memory and cognitive function may be helped by its ability to defend against oxidative stress in the brain, reduce inflammation, and enhance blood flow, all of which are factors that contribute to brain health.
Elderberry has been shown to enhance athletic performance and may help to reduce fatigue and improve endurance. It is possible that the antioxidant capabilities of this substance will assist in lowering the levels of oxidative stress and inflammation in the body, both of which can contribute to fatigue and injury to the muscles. There is evidence that elderberry has a number of positive effects on the quality of sleep. It can assist in lowering inflammation, enhancing blood flow, and production of melatonin, all of which can help to improve the quality of sleep as well as the amount of time spent sleeping.

Elderberry is usually thought to be safe for consumption when ingested in moderate doses; nevertheless, there are some restrictions on how it can be used. It is important to exercise caution when taking elderberry supplements because they have the potential to interact negatively with certain drugs, including immunosuppressants and diuretics. Elderberry is something that should probably be avoided by individuals who suffer from autoimmune illnesses or allergies to plants in the honeysuckle family. Elderberries that have not yet reached maturity as well as other components of the plant, such as the leaves and stems, are poisonous and should not be consumed.

A plant with medical benefits, licorice, also known as Glycyrrhiza glabra, has been used for ages. Although it was originally from Europe and Asia, it has since become naturalized in a great many other regions across the globe. Licorice is loaded with a number of bioactive components, such as glycyrrhizin, flavonoids, and polysaccharides, all of which have been linked to a variety of positive effects on human health.

The therapeutic benefits of licorice are due to the presence of a number of compounds within the licorice root. The unique flavor of licorice root is due to a compound called glycyrrhizin, which has a pleasant sweetness to it and can be found in the licorice root. It has been demonstrated to possess a variety of beneficial effects for one's health, such as anti-inflammatory, antiviral, and antioxidant qualities.

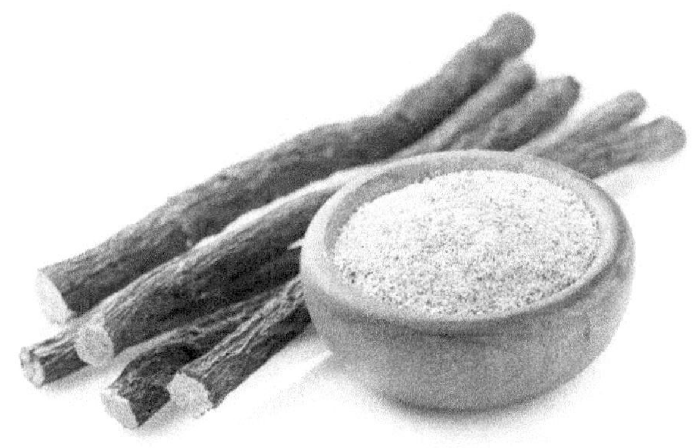

Licorice contains flavonoids such as liquiritin and isoliquiritin, both of which have been proven to possess antioxidant, anti-inflammatory, and antiviral properties. Licorice is also an ingredient in candy called anise. Licorice contains polysaccharides, some of which have been demonstrated to modulate the immune system. One example of this is glycyrrhizic acid, which may be found in licorice.

Licorice has been traditionally used for its medicinal properties, and modern research has confirmed many of its traditional uses. Licorice can be obtained in a number of different preparations, such as licorice supplements, licorice tea, and licorice extract.

Historically, licorice has been employed as a remedy for a variety of respiratory conditions, including coughs and bronchitis. It has been demonstrated to possess expectorant characteristics, which aid to break up phlegm and mucus in the respiratory tract so that they can be expelled more easily.
Historically, licorice has been employed as a remedy for a variety of digestive conditions, including indigestion, acid reflux, and stomach ulcers. It has been established that it possesses anti-inflammatory qualities, which make it capable of assisting in the reduction of inflammation that occurs in the digestive tract.
It has been demonstrated that licorice can improve immune function by boosting the activity of immune cells such natural killer cells and T cells.

Historically, licorice has been utilized in the treatment of a variety of skin disorders, including eczema and psoriasis. It has been shown to have anti-inflammatory and antioxidant properties, which can help to reduce inflammation and protect against oxidative stress in the skin.

It has been demonstrated that licorice possesses adaptogenic qualities, which make it useful in the treatment of anxiety and stress. Levels of the stress hormone cortisol, which if left unchecked, can contribute to feelings of tension and worry, may be regulated by this.

It has been proven that licorice contains antiviral characteristics, and these features may assist in the treatment of a variety of viral illnesses. These infections include herpes simplex virus, human immunodeficiency virus (HIV), and hepatitis C virus.

It has been demonstrated that licorice contains a number of possible anticancer qualities, and these features may assist to prevent the emergence of a variety of cancer forms, including breast, colon, and prostate cancer.
It has been demonstrated that licorice offers a number of possible benefits for cognitive function. Memory and attention are two areas that can benefit from its use, as well as the prevention of cognitive deterioration associated with aging.

It has been demonstrated that licorice offers a number of potential benefits for the modulation of hormones. It can help to regulate cortisol levels, which can contribute to feelings of stress and anxiety, and may also help to regulate estrogen levels in women.

It has been demonstrated that licorice offers a number of possible benefits for the healing of wounds. It has been shown to have anti-inflammatory as well as antioxidant qualities, both of which can assist in bringing about a reduction in inflammation and a hastening of the healing process in the skin.

Licorice may have some positive effects on health, but there are also some potential drawbacks and safety concerns that should be taken into consideration. When ingested in excessive quantities, the component known as glycyrrhizin that is found in licorice can lead to a number of adverse effects, some of which include hypertension, hypokalemia, and edema. As a result, licorice supplements must to be utilized with extreme caution, and individuals who suffer from conditions such as high blood pressure, heart disease, or kidney illness ought to steer clear of licorice supplements altogether. Licorice has the potential to interact negatively with a number of drugs, including corticosteroids and diuretics; therefore, it must be used with extreme caution in patients who are already on these treatments.

Ginger is a spice that has been utilized for hundreds of years due to the therapeutic benefits it offers. It is native to Southeast Asia, but has since been naturalized in many other parts of the world. Ginger contains a variety of compounds, such as gingerols, shogaols, and zingerone, all of which have been demonstrated to be beneficial to one's health in a variety of different ways.

Ginger is known to have a variety of health benefits due to the presence of several chemicals within the root. Gingerols are a group of chemicals that are responsible for the pungent taste of ginger. These compounds have also been found to have various potential health advantages, including anti-inflammatory and antioxidant effects.

Ginger is a root that comes from the ginger plant. It has been demonstrated that shogaols, a different set of chemicals that are generated when ginger is dried or cooked, possess more potent anti-inflammatory and antioxidant activities than gingerols. Zingerone is a chemical that is responsible for the aroma of ginger and has been proven to offer various potential health advantages, including anti-inflammatory and antifungal effects. Zingerone is also responsible for the aroma of ginger.

Ginger has a long history of usage in traditional medicine, and recent research has supported many of the medical purposes that ginger has traditionally been put to. It is available in several forms, including ginger supplements, ginger tea, and ginger extract.

Ginger has been proven to be useful in reducing nausea and vomiting caused by a variety of illnesses, including morning sickness, chemotherapy-induced nausea, and postoperative nausea and vomiting. This is due to ginger's ability to stimulate the body's release of serotonin, which in turn reduces feelings of nausea and vomiting.
Ginger is known to possess anti-inflammatory qualities, and these features may help reduce inflammation and pain associated with a number of disorders. These conditions include osteoarthritis, rheumatoid arthritis, and menstruation discomfort.

Ginger has been demonstrated to provide potential advantages for heart health by helping to lower cholesterol levels and control blood sugar levels. These benefits can be attributed to ginger's anti-inflammatory and blood sugar regulating properties.

Ginger has been used medicinally for the treatment of respiratory illnesses like colds and the flu since ancient times. It has been demonstrated to possess expectorant characteristics, which aid to break up phlegm and mucus in the respiratory tract so that they can be expelled more easily.

It has been demonstrated that ginger may offer a number of possible benefits for digestive health. It can be beneficial for digestion in that it can assist to increase digestion, reduce bloating and flatulence, and it may also be beneficial for protecting against stomach ulcers.

Ginger has been shown to have potential benefits for treating migraines. By lowering inflammation and bringing neurotransmitter levels in the brain back under control, it can make migraines less severe and less frequent for those who suffer from them.

It has been demonstrated that ginger possesses a number of possible anticancer qualities, and these features may assist to prevent the development of a number of different types of cancer, including colon, ovarian, and pancreatic cancer.

There is some evidence that ginger may have a number of positive effects on cognitive performance. Memory and attention are two areas that can benefit from its use, as well as the prevention of cognitive deterioration associated with aging.

It has been demonstrated that ginger may be useful in treating erectile dysfunction by increasing the amount of blood that flows to the penis and increasing the amount of nitric oxide that is produced by the body.
It has been demonstrated that ginger may have various possible benefits for the performance of athletes. It has been shown to be effective in reducing inflammation and

muscular pain, and it may also aid improve endurance and speed.

Ginger may have some positive effects on your health, but there are also some potential drawbacks and safety concerns you should be aware of. Ginger supplements may interact with certain medications, such as blood thinners and diabetes medications, and should be used with caution. When ingested in high quantities, ginger has the potential to induce a number of moderate adverse effects, including heartburn and stomach discomfort. Andrographis is a plant that has been used for medicinal purposes for a number of centuries in traditional medicine due to the potential health benefits that it offers. Although it was originally from India and Sri Lanka, it has since become naturalized in a number of different regions across the globe. Andrographis includes a number of compounds, one of which is called andrographolide, which research has shown to have a variety of possible positive effects on human health.

Andrographis is made up of a number of different compounds, each of which contributes to the plant's unique medical qualities. Andrographolide is a chemical that is present in Andrographis in high concentrations. It has been demonstrated to offer a number of possible health advantages, including anti-inflammatory, antioxidant, and antiviral characteristics. Andrographolide is also responsible for the bitter taste of Andrographis.

Andrographis has a long history of usage in traditional medicine, and recent study has supported many of the therapeutic applications that have traditionally been attributed to it. Andrographis is offered in a variety of formats, including as dietary supplements, infusions, and teas. It is also accessible as a standalone extract.

Andrographis has a long history of use as a remedy for a variety of respiratory conditions, including the common cold, influenza, and bronchitis. It has been demonstrated to have the potential for a variety of advantages, including a reduction in the intensity and duration of respiratory infections, as well as an improvement in immunological function.

Andrographis has been demonstrated to have anti-inflammatory qualities, and it may help to lessen the inflammation and pain associated with a number of illnesses, such as inflammatory bowel disease, rheumatoid arthritis, and osteoarthritis.

It has been demonstrated that andrographis has a number of potential benefits for the digestive function. It can be beneficial for digestion in that it can assist to increase digestion, reduce bloating and flatulence, and it may also be beneficial for protecting against stomach ulcers.

Andrographis has a long history of use as a medicinal remedy for a variety of liver conditions, including hepatitis and cirrhosis. It has been shown to have potential benefits for reducing liver damage and enhancing liver function.

Andrographis showed promise as a possible treatment for a number of skin conditions, including acne, eczema, and psoriasis, according to recent research. It can be beneficial in reducing inflammation and assisting in the healing process of the skin.

Andrographis has showed promise as a therapeutic agent for a variety of viral diseases, including HIV, influenza, and dengue fever. It has the potential to improve immunological function while also inhibiting the replication of viruses.

Andrographis has been proven to possess a number of possible anticancer characteristics, and it may help to prevent the development of a variety of cancers, including cancer of the liver, cancer of the colon, and cancer of the prostate.

Andrographis has been demonstrated to have a number of possible benefits for the cognitive function of the body. Memory and attention are two areas that can benefit from its use, as well as the prevention of cognitive deterioration associated with aging.

Andrographis has showed promise as a treatment option for patients with type 2 diabetes who are looking for ways to better control their blood sugar levels. It can aid in enhancing insulin sensitivity and lowering inflammatory responses in the body.

It has been demonstrated that andrographis may have prospective benefits for increasing the cardiovascular system's health. It is possible for it to assist in bringing down blood pressure, lessening inflammation in the arteries, and bettering lipid profiles.

Andrographis may have some positive effects on health, but there are also some potential drawbacks and safety concerns that should be taken into consideration. Andrographis supplements may interfere with some medications, including those used to treat diabetes and blood thinners; therefore, they should be used with caution if you are already on any of these medications.

Andrographis can have adverse effects in certain individuals, including nausea, diarrhea, and allergic responses. This is particularly common in children. If you have a medical problem or are taking medication, it is essential to discuss the use of andrographis pills or extract with a qualified medical professional prior to beginning treatment with either option.

Olive trees, or Olea europaea as they are more formally known in the scientific community, are a species of tree that are native to the Mediterranean region. Olive leaf is the leaf of the olive tree. Olive leaf has been used for centuries for its potential health benefits and is known to contain several compounds, including oleuropein, that have been shown to have several potential health benefits.

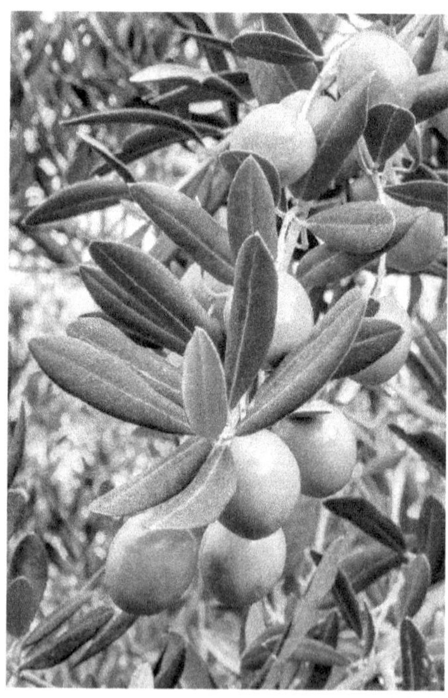

Olive leaf includes a number of different compounds, each of which may contribute to the olive leaf's unique health benefits. Oleuropein is a compound that may be found in olive leaf in high amounts. It has been demonstrated to have numerous possible health benefits, such as anti-inflammatory, antioxidant, and antibacterial characteristics. Flavonoids, secoiridoids, and phenolic acids are some of the other substances that can be found in olive leaves.

Olive leaf has a long history of use for its therapeutic qualities, and recent scientific research has validated a number of the traditional use of olive leaf. Olive leaf can be consumed in a number of different ways, such as in the form of olive leaf supplements, olive leaf tea, and olive leaf extract.

Olive leaf has been proven to have anti-inflammatory qualities and may help reduce inflammation associated with a number of illnesses, including arthritis, asthma, and inflammatory bowel disease.

Olive leaf has been shown to have potential benefits for lowering cholesterol levels in the blood. It has been shown to be effective in lowering LDL cholesterol levels while simultaneously raising HDL cholesterol levels, which may assist in lowering the risk of developing cardiovascular disease.

Olive leaf extract has showed promise as a possible immune-boosting agent, according to a number of scientific studies. It is possible that it will assist boost the development of white blood cells, which are the cells in the blood that are responsible for warding off infections and disorders.

It has been demonstrated that olive leaf could potentially be beneficial in the treatment of a variety of illnesses, including bacterial and viral infections. It has the potential to prevent the multiplication of dangerous bacteria and viruses, including those that are responsible for respiratory infections and gastroenteritis.

Olive leaf extract has showed promise as a possible diabetes management aid, according to recent research. It is possible for it to help minimize the chance of developing type 2 diabetes by lowering blood sugar levels and improving insulin sensitivity.

Olive leaf has been proven to have a number of possible anticancer qualities, and it may help to guard against the development of a number of different types of cancer, including breast, colon, and prostate cancer.

Olive leaf has been demonstrated to have the capacity to protect against neurodegenerative disorders including Alzheimer's disease and Parkinson's disease. It has the potential to defend against inflammation and neuronal damage, as well as assist lessen the effects of oxidative stress in the brain.

It has been demonstrated that olive leaf may have potential benefits for enhancing the health of the skin. It can assist in minimizing inflammation and protect against oxidative stress in the skin, both of which can help to enhance the appearance of the skin and may help to minimize the chance of developing skin cancer.

Olive leaf extract has been proven to have possible health advantages, including the prevention of heart disease. It can assist in the reduction of arterial inflammation as well as oxidative stress, and also in the lowering of blood pressure and the improvement of lipid profiles.

Olive leaf has been demonstrated to have potential benefits for boosting bone health, and this includes the prevention of bone loss. It is possible for it to assist in the process of increasing bone mineral density and lowering the risk of osteoporosis.

While olive leaf has several potential health benefits, there are some limitations and precautions to consider. Olive leaf supplements have the potential to interact negatively with a variety of medications, including those for the treatment of diabetes and blood thinners; as a result, their usage in these scenarios is strongly discouraged. Olive leaf extract has been linked in several studies to a variety of adverse effects, including diarrhea and allergic responses. If you have a medical problem or are taking medication, it is essential to discuss the use of olive leaf supplements or extract with a qualified medical professional prior to beginning treatment with either option.

St. John's Wort, also known as Hypericum perforatum, is a plant that has a long history of use as a therapeutic remedy due to the possible benefits it offers to one's health. Although it was originally from Europe, it is currently produced and grown in many countries all over the world. The possible health advantages of St. John's Wort are due to the presence of a number of compounds within the plant, the most notable of which are hypericin and hyperforin.

St. John's Wort contains several compounds that are responsible for its potential health benefits. Both hypericin and hyperforin are two substances that are found in high concentrations in St. John's Wort. These compounds have been demonstrated to have a number of possible health advantages, and their presence in the plant is responsible for their high concentrations. Other compounds found in St. John's Wort include flavonoids, xanthones, and catechins.

St. John's Wort has been used traditionally for its therapeutic benefits, and research conducted in more recent times has verified many of the traditional uses of the herb. St. John's Wort is available in several forms, including St. John's Wort supplements, St. John's Wort tea, and St. John's Wort extract.

It has been demonstrated that the use of St. John's Wort as a potential treatment for mild to moderate depression may be beneficial. The levels of the neurotransmitters serotonin, dopamine, and noradrenaline, which are related with the regulation of mood, can be helped to increase by using this technique.

It has been demonstrated that the herb St. John's Wort may be beneficial for reducing feelings of anxiety. It has the potential to assist in the alleviation of stressful and tense feelings and the promotion of relaxation.

St. John's Wort has been traditionally used for treating skin conditions, including wounds, burns, and insect bites. It may aid in the reduction of inflammation and the speeding up of wound healing.

It has been demonstrated that St. John's Wort may be beneficial in the treatment of menopausal symptoms, such as hot flashes and irritability fluctuations. It may assist in restoring a healthy hormonal balance and lessening the severity of symptoms associated with the menopause.

It has been shown that the herb St. John's Wort may have the ability to improve cognitive function in a variety of ways, including memory and concentration. It has the potential to assist in enhancing brain cell function as well as blood flow to the brain.

It has been proven that St. John's Wort may be useful in the treatment of seasonal affective disorder (SAD), a form of depression that is brought on by the change in seasons. It has been shown to be helpful in regulating the levels of neurotransmitters that are related with the control of mood, as well as in reducing the symptoms of depression associated with SAD.

St. John's Wort has been shown to have potential benefits for protecting against neurodegenerative diseases, such as Alzheimer's and Parkinson's disease. It has the potential to help reduce inflammation and oxidative stress in the brain, as well as protect neurons from being damaged.

Obsessive-compulsive disorder (OCD) is an anxiety illness that can be treated with St. John's Wort, which has been found to have potential advantages. It may be helpful in reducing OCD symptoms, such as obsessive behaviors and repetitive thoughts, which can be caused by the condition.

St. John's Wort has been proven to have potential benefits for alleviating nerve pain, including sciatica and neuropathic pain. This includes the pain associated with diabetic neuropathy. It can assist in lowering inflammation and facilitating the regeneration of nerves.

It has been demonstrated that the herb St. John's Wort may have potential benefits for improving immunological function. It is possible that it will assist boost the development of white blood cells, which are the cells in the blood that are responsible for warding off infections and disorders.

Although there is some evidence that St. John's Wort could be beneficial to one's health, it is essential to consume the herb with extreme caution and only after seeing a qualified medical professional. St. John's Wort can interact with several medications, including antidepressants, birth control pills, and blood thinners. It is also possible for it to induce adverse effects such as dry mouth, light sensitivity, and dizziness.

When it comes to the prevention and treatment of viral infections, herbal antivirals present a promising alternative or supplementary therapy option. They have the potential to provide a number of benefits, including as a lower risk of adverse effects, improved immune system function, cost-effective antiviral action, and tailored antiviral activity. In addition, a variety of herbal antivirals have been demonstrated to be effective against a wide variety of viruses, which enables them to serve as a flexible and potentially beneficial instrument in the prevention and treatment of viral infections.

Herbal antivirals also have some limitations. To begin, it is possible that their efficacy has not been as thoroughly researched as that of standard antiviral drugs, which have been put through a significant amount of clinical testing. Second, because the FDA does not control herbal medicines, there is a possibility that they have been tampered with or contaminated in some way. Third, there is a possibility that certain individuals will have allergic responses or other negative effects when they use herbal treatments. It is also important to note that the effectiveness of herbal antivirals can vary depending on several factors, including the type of virus being targeted, the stage of the infection, and the individual's overall health and immune system function.

Importance of using herbal antivirals in conjunction with other treatments

As individuals search for non-traditional approaches to the prevention and treatment of viral infections, the use of herbal antivirals is becoming an increasingly common practice. Even though herbal antivirals may have some positive effects, it is essential to keep in mind that they are not intended to take the place of conventional medicines in any way. In this section, we will talk about the significance of taking herbal antivirals in conjunction with other types of treatment.

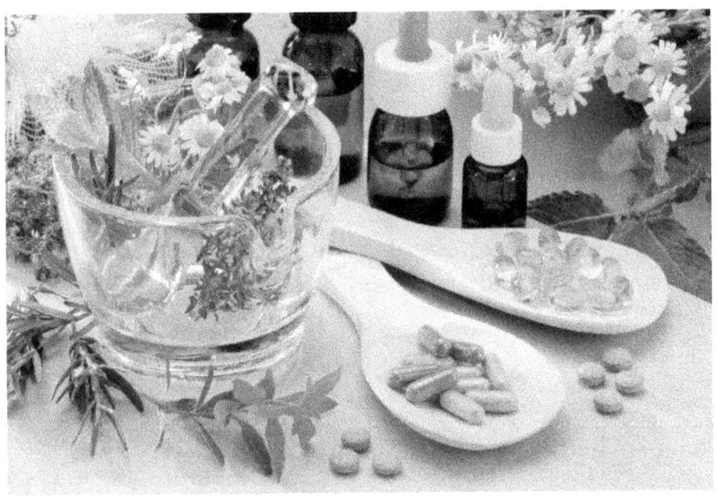

Herbal antivirals have the potential to provide a number of health benefits, including the enhancement of immune function, reduction of inflammatory response, and the elimination of viral infections. They are frequently utilized as a non-pharmaceutical alternative to conventional medicines, which frequently come with a plethora of potential adverse effects and may not be effective against all forms of viral infections.

Supplements, teas, and extracts are some of the forms in which herbal antivirals can be taken to combat viral infections. They are often less expensive than conventional medications and are more readily available.

Even while herbal antivirals have the potential to be beneficial, it is essential to remember that in order for them to be effective, they must be used in conjunction with other treatments. Here are a few explanations:
Infections caused by viruses can range from being relatively harmless to being life-threatening, and depending on the severity of the illness, traditional medical treatment may be required in order to prevent complications and expedite the healing process. Even while herbal antivirals have the potential to be beneficial, it's possible that they won't be enough to treat serious infections.
Antiviral pharmaceuticals are treatments that target the virus itself in order to treat viral infections. These medications can be used to treat viral infections. They accomplish this by preventing the virus from multiplying and from spreading to other parts of the body. Antiviral medication is often used for the treatment of more serious viral infections, such as HIV, hepatitis B and C, and the flu.
While herbal antivirals can be effective in boosting the immune system and fighting against viral infections, they may not be sufficient for severe infections. In these circumstances, the treatment of the infection and the prevention of consequences may need the use of antiviral drugs.
Vaccinations are a form of preventative medicine that can be of assistance in warding off diseases caused by

viruses. In order to be effective, they act by inducing the body's immune system to produce antibodies that are effective against certain viruses. These antibodies can either help avoid infection or lessen the severity of symptoms.

Even though herbal antivirals have the potential to be beneficial for preventing viral infections, it is possible that they are not effective enough to treat all strains of viruses. When it comes to the prevention of some viral illnesses, such as influenza, hepatitis B, and human papillomavirus (HPV), vaccines can offer a method that is both more focused and more successful.

Treatments that can help to reduce symptoms and promote the body's natural healing processes are what are meant to fall under the category of "supportive care." This can consist of things like rest, water, pain relief, and nutrition, among other things.

While herbal antivirals can help to boost the immune system and fight against viral infections, they may not be sufficient for addressing the symptoms associated with severe infections. Supportive care can assist with the management of symptoms and the promotion of recovery, both of which are extremely important in reducing the risk of complications and improving overall health.

Combination therapy is a method of treating a patient with more than one treatment at the same time or in a certain order in order to get better results than would be possible with a single treatment alone. Combination therapy can be especially helpful in the setting of viral infections because it can both avoid viral resistance and enhance the effectiveness of individual treatments. In this section, we will examine the importance of utilizing herbal antivirals in conjunction with other therapies and why it may be more successful to use combination therapy for treating viral infections.

Combination therapy has a number of significant benefits, one of the most significant of which is its capacity to avoid viral resistance. When a virus undergoes a mutation as a defense mechanism against a treatment, this phenomenon is known as viral resistance. Using multiple treatments that target different aspects of the virus can reduce the likelihood of viral resistance.

Combination therapy may be used, for instance, in the treatment of hepatitis C. This type of treatment may involve the use of multiple antiviral drugs that attack various stages of the life cycle of the virus. This strategy may lessen the likelihood of the virus developing resistance and raise the probability of achieving a sustained virologic response, also known as SVR. SVR is defined as the absence of detectable virus in the blood six months after treatment has been administered.

Combination therapy can also enhance the effectiveness of individual treatments. It's possible for multiple treatments to act together to provide a synergistic effect, which simply means that the overall benefit is bigger than the sum of the effects produced by each treatment on its own.

For instance, a study that was published in the Journal of Ethnopharmacology indicated that treating influenza with a combination of zanamivir (a conventional antiviral medicine) and andrographis paniculata was more effective than treating the illness with either of the treatments individually. The combination of Andrographis paniculata and zanamivir resulted in a greater reduction in viral load and more rapid recovery from symptoms.

It is possible that using numerous therapies will help lessen the adverse effects that are caused by each particular treatment. Some conventional therapies for viral infections can induce major adverse effects, such as nausea, vomiting, and exhaustion. These symptoms can sometimes even be life threatening. It is feasible that the dose of each therapy may be decreased if numerous treatments were combined into one. This would result in fewer adverse effects.

The term "synergistic effects" refers to the phenomenon in which the combined effect of two or more therapies is higher than the total of the effects produced by each therapy individually. When it comes to fighting viral infections, taking various therapies at the same time can cause synergistic effects, which can increase the efficiency of each individual treatment. In this section, we will explore the significance of synergistic effects in the treatment of viral infections as well as the advantages of utilizing herbal antivirals in conjunction with other treatments.

It is possible to increase the overall efficacy of each treatment by combining medicines that work through distinct modes of action. For example, combining an antiviral medication with an immunomodulator can enhance the immune system's response to the virus and improve the antiviral effect of the medication.
According to the findings of a study that was published in the Journal of Medical Virology, treating hepatitis C with a combination of the antiviral medicine ribavirin and the immunomodulator interferon-alpha was more effective than treating the condition with either treatment alone. The combination therapy resulted in a higher rate of sustained virologic response (SVR), which is the absence of detectable virus in the blood six months after

treatment. This is the gold standard for measuring treatment success.

It is possible to lessen the likelihood of the virus developing resistance by utilizing numerous therapies that attack the infection from a variety of angles. When a virus undergoes a mutation as a defense mechanism against a treatment, this phenomenon is known as viral resistance. It is less probable that the virus will develop resistance to all of the treatments if many therapies are used, each of which targets a distinct stage of the life cycle of the virus.

For example, combination therapy for HIV may involve using a combination of antiretroviral drugs that focus on several viral life cycle stages. This strategy may raise the possibility of long-term viral suppression while simultaneously decreasing the danger that viruses will develop resistance to the treatment.

Using a combination of treatments rather than just one can help reduce the negative effects that each treatment may have. Some conventional therapies for viral infections can induce major adverse effects, such as nausea, vomiting, and exhaustion. These symptoms can sometimes even be life threatening. It is feasible that the dose of each therapy may be decreased if numerous treatments were combined into one.

Since ancient times, individuals have turned to herbal antivirals as a treatment for viral illnesses. They are frequently believed to be a natural alternative to traditional antiviral medications, which could have undesirable side effects and might even contribute to the evolution of viruses that are resistant to certain drugs. In recent years, research has indicated that herbal antivirals may have a role in improving immune function. This improvement in immune function can assist to prevent and treat viral infections. In this essay, we will discuss how herbal antivirals may enhance immune function and why this is an important reason to use them in conjunction with other treatments for viral infections.

Herbal antivirals are effective because they target several stages of the viral replication process. For example, they prevent viruses from entering host cells, they stop viruses from replicating, and they boost immune function. By boosting immune function, one of the most significant ways in which herbal antivirals may be effective in the treatment of viral infections is one of the ways in which they may be beneficial overall. It has been demonstrated that certain herbal antivirals can boost the immune system. This can assist in the prevention of viral infections and improve the body's ability to fight against viral infections.

Echinacea, for instance, has been proven to enhance the activity of immune cells such as macrophages and natural killer cells. These cells are important for recognizing and eliminating viruses in the body. Garlic includes chemicals that can stimulate the activity of immune cells and promote the creation of antibodies, both of which assist to kill viruses. Garlic has been used for centuries as a traditional remedy for a wide range of ailments. Andrographis has been shown to stimulate the production of interferon, which is a protein that helps to prevent viral replication and spread.

It has been demonstrated that several herbal antivirals, in addition to boosting the immune system, also have antioxidant and anti-inflammatory benefits. Antioxidants have been shown to be effective in lowering oxidative stress as well as inflammation, both of which are linked to viral infections. Herbal antivirals can help to boost the body's ability to fight off viruses by improving immune function and reducing oxidative stress and inflammation.

The traditional medical therapies for viral infections can come with a variety of unpleasant side effects, such as gastrointestinal distress, headaches, and nausea. These unwanted consequences can be distressing, and they might even cause the patient to stop receiving treatment. When used with conventional treatments, herbal antivirals, on the other hand, have the potential to lessen the severity of some of these adverse effects.

When treating viral infections, conventional medicines are typically used in conjunction with herbal antivirals as a complimentary therapy. They accomplish their goals by inhibiting specific stages of viral replication and boosting immune function, both of which contribute to lowering the risk of viral infections and speeding up their treatment. Herbal antivirals, when combined with traditional medical therapies, have the potential to offer a more all-encompassing and fruitful treatment strategy for viral infections.

Antiviral drugs and other conventional therapies for viral infections, such antibiotics, sometimes come with undesirable side effects. These unwanted consequences can range from somewhat harmless, such as gastrointestinal distress, to quite harmful, such as poisoning to the liver. It is possible for the adverse effects of conventional treatments to be so severe that the patient is forced to stop receiving therapy altogether in some instances.

Herbal antivirals could be able to mitigate some of the negative effects that come along with using traditional medicines to treat viral infections. For example, some herbal antivirals may be less likely to cause gastrointestinal upset or liver toxicity than conventional antiviral medications. Herbal antivirals may enhance adherence to treatment and reduce the overall burden of viral infections since they lessen the likelihood of experiencing adverse effects.

It has been demonstrated that garlic, a common herbal antiviral, can lessen the negative effects that are associated with conventional antiviral drugs. Patients who took garlic in conjunction with traditional antiviral treatment saw fewer adverse effects, such as diarrhea and abdominal pain, in comparison to patients who only took the conventional medication. This hints that garlic may be able to assist decrease the adverse effects on the digestive tract that are associated with traditional antiviral drugs.

Ginger is another another antiviral herbal remedy that has the potential to mitigate the negative effects of conventional medicines. Ginger has been demonstrated to have anti-inflammatory effects, which means that it can help to lessen the inflammation that is linked with viral infections as well as the negative effects of traditional therapies. In addition, ginger has been shown to have anti-nausea effects, which may help to reduce the nausea associated with some antiviral medications.

Another herbal antiviral that may help lessen the negative effects of conventional medicines is licorice, which can be purchased online. It has been demonstrated that licorice has anti-inflammatory actions, which can help to lessen the inflammation caused by viral infections as well as the negative effects of traditional treatments. In addition, research has revealed that licorice has hepatoprotective properties, which means that it can help protect the liver from the harm that may be caused by using some antiviral drugs.

Combination treatments for viral infections may benefit from the use of herbal antivirals as an additional component. Using herbal antivirals in conjunction with conventional therapies can be beneficial for a number of reasons, including the following:

The immune system can be strengthened with the help of herbal antivirals, which can be of use in both the prevention of and the treatment of viral infections. Herbal antivirals, when used in conjunction with conventional therapies, have the potential to boost the immune system's capacity to fight against viral infections.

It's possible that certain herbal antivirals can help lessen the discomfort caused by conventional therapies. For example, a study published in the journal BMC Complementary and Alternative Medicine found that a combination of milk thistle and interferon-alpha (a conventional treatment for hepatitis C) reduced the side effects of interferon-alpha.

In conjunction with conventional therapies, the use of herbal antivirals may assist to decrease side effects, which in turn may enhance general quality of life and aid recovery.

It is possible that the use of certain herbal antivirals in conjunction with conventional treatments will result in synergistic effects. For instance, a study that was published in the Journal of Ethnopharmacology indicated that treating influenza with a combination of zanamivir (a conventional antiviral medicine) and andrographis paniculata was more effective than treating the illness with either of the treatments individually.

The use of herbal antivirals in conjunction with conventional treatments has the potential to help improve the efficacy of both treatments, which in turn may result in improved outcomes for the patient.

In conclusion, herbal antivirals have the potential to be beneficial in both the prevention of viral infections and the treatment of viral infections; however, they should be used in conjunction with other treatments. Conventional treatments may be necessary for severe infections, and combination therapy may be more effective than using either treatment alone. Herbal antivirals may have additive effects, improve immune function, and assist in mitigating the negative effects of conventional medicines. Before combining herbal antivirals with other therapies, it is essential to discuss your treatment plan with a medical professional to see whether or not the combination will be both beneficial and risk-free for your circumstances.

CHAPTER III

Top Herbal Antivirals for Building Resilience

An overview of the most potent herbal antivirals for boosting resistance to viral threats

For ages, viral infections have been prevented and treated with herbal antivirals. These organic treatments can improve immunological response, lessen the intensity and length of symptoms, and aid in avoiding viral infections. The best herbal antivirals for boosting resistance to viral threats will be briefly discussed in this section.

Echinacea is a popular herbal antiviral that has been utilized for preventing and treating viral infections for ages. In addition to improving immunological function, it also lessens the intensity and duration of symptoms. The body's main line of defense against viral infections is the white blood cell, which is stimulated by substances found in echinacea.

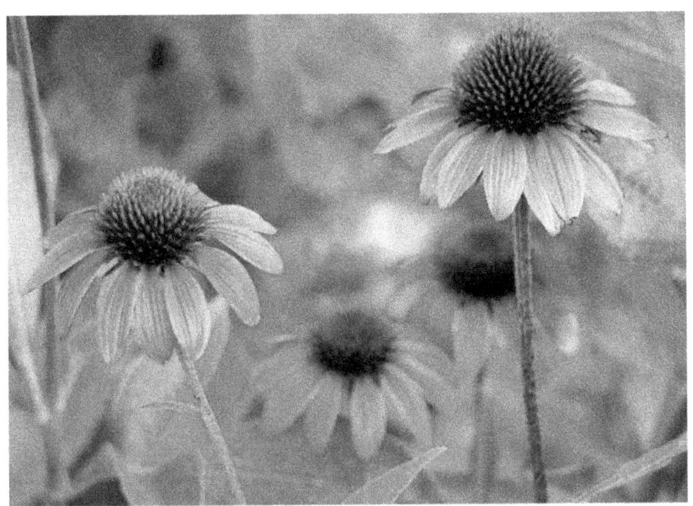

Another effective natural antiviral used for ages to both prevent and treat viral infections is garlic. There are substances in garlic that have been demonstrated to be antiviral, antibacterial, and antifungal. Additionally, garlic can improve immune response and lessen the intensity and duration of symptoms.

For centuries, individuals have used elderberry, a well-known natural antiviral, to prevent and treat viral infections, including the flu. Elderberries include substances that have been demonstrated to have antiviral effects and can boost immune system performance. Elderberry has been demonstrated to lessen the severity and persistence of flu symptoms, and it may even contribute to its prevention.

Licorice is a powerful herbal antiviral that has been used for centuries to prevent and treat viral infections. There are substances in licorice that have been found to be antiviral, antibacterial, and anti-inflammatory. Licorice can improve immunological response, as well as lessen the intensity and duration of symptoms. Additionally, it might aid in avoiding viral infections.

A lesser-known herbal antiviral called andrographis has been used for many years to both prevent and treat viral infections. Compounds found in andrographis have been demonstrated to have antiviral, antibacterial, and anti-inflammatory effects. The immune system can be strengthened by andrographis, which can also lessen symptom intensity and duration. Additionally, it might aid in avoiding viral infections.

In summary, herbal antivirals can be useful agents for boosting resistance to viral dangers. For preventing and treating viral infections, some of the most potent herbal antivirals include echinacea, garlic, elderberry, licorice, and andrographis. These organic treatments can improve immunological response, lessen the intensity and length of symptoms, and aid in avoiding viral infections. Herbal antivirals can mix with other medications and have potential negative effects, therefore it is crucial to discuss their use with a healthcare professional before using.

How each herbal antiviral works and its benefits

Since ancient times, the plant echinacea has been used to cure a wide range of illnesses, including the common cold, the flu, and other viral diseases. It is well known for its ability to fight viruses and strengthen the immune system. We will examine echinacea's antiviral properties and potential advantages in this section.

Numerous substances found in echinacea have been demonstrated to have antiviral effects. The most well-known of these substances are alkamides, echinacoside, and echinacin. Echinacea is a strong herbal antiviral due to the interaction of these chemicals, which prevent the replication of viruses.

Studies have shown that echinacea can inhibit the replication of a variety of viruses, including influenza, herpes simplex virus, and respiratory syncytial virus. Echinacea accomplishes this by promoting the development of white blood cells, the body's main line of defense against infections.
There are a number of possible advantages for echinacea as an antiviral. Some of these benefits include:
It has been demonstrated that echinacea improves immunological function, aiding the body in warding against viral illnesses. The body's main line of defense against infections is the white blood cell, which is stimulated by echinacea.

It has been demonstrated that echinacea lessens the intensity and persistence of viral infection-related symptoms. Echinacea has been found in studies to shorten the length and intensity of cold and flu symptoms.
In order to increase resistance against viral threats without running the danger of the negative side effects associated with traditional therapies, echinacea is a safe and natural cure. Echinacea has been shown to have broad spectrum antiviral activity, meaning it can inhibit the replication of a variety of viruses. Echinacea is an affordable treatment that is widely accessible in most health food stores and is simple to use in a balanced diet.
Since ancient times, individuals have taken advantage of the healing powers of garlic, a common culinary herb. It has been demonstrated to provide a number of health advantages, including lowering blood pressure, reducing

inflammation, and raising cholesterol levels. It has been proven that the herbal antiviral power of garlic increases resistance to viral dangers. We will explore garlic's antiviral properties and potential advantages in this section.

Numerous substances found in garlic have been demonstrated to have antiviral effects. Allicin, the most well-known of these substances, is released when garlic is chopped or crushed. Numerous antimicrobial characteristics of allicin, such as antiviral, antibacterial, and antifungal activity, have been demonstrated.
Studies have shown that allicin can inhibit the replication of a variety of viruses, including the herpes simplex virus, HIV, and the influenza virus. Allicin accomplishes this by obstructing the virus' capacity to multiply and infect cells. Ajoene, alliin, and allixin are some of the other antiviral substances found in garlic in addition to allicin. Together, these substances give garlic its powerful antiviral capabilities.
As an antiviral, garlic has been demonstrated to have a number of potential advantages. Some of these benefits include:

The immune system can be strengthened by garlic, which can aid the body in warding against viral illnesses. White blood cells, the body's main line of defense against infections, are stimulated by garlic.
It has been demonstrated that garlic can lessen the intensity and persistence of viral infection-related symptoms. Garlic can lessen the intensity of cold and flu symptoms and may even help to prevent these infections from starting in the first place, according to studies.

Garlic is a safe and natural remedy that can be used to enhance resistance to viral threats without the risk of harmful side effects associated with conventional treatments.

It has been demonstrated that garlic has broad spectrum antiviral activity, which means that it can prevent the replication of numerous viruses. Most grocery stores carry garlic, which is an affordable treatment that is simple to include in a balanced diet.

In addition to the common cold, flu, and other viral infections, elderberry is a well-known herbal treatment that has been used for millennia to cure a number of illnesses. It is well known for its ability to fight viruses and strengthen the immune system. This section will examine elderberry's antiviral properties and potential advantages.

Numerous substances found in elderberries have been demonstrated to have antiviral effects. Anthocyanins, flavonoids, and phenolic acids are the most popular forms of these substances. These compounds work together to inhibit the replication of viruses, making elderberry a potent herbal antiviral.

According to studies, elderberry can stop the spread of a number of viruses, including the herpes simplex virus (HSV), the influenza virus, and the human immunodeficiency virus (HIV). This is accomplished by elderberry by encouraging the synthesis of cytokines, which are proteins that assist in controlling the immune response and lowering inflammation.

There are a number of possible advantages of elderberry as an antiviral. Some of these benefits include:

Elderberry has been demonstrated to boost immunological response, which may aid the body in fighting off viral infections. Inflammation is reduced and the immune system is better controlled when cytokines are produced as a result of elderberry.

It has been demonstrated that elderberry can lessen the intensity and duration of viral infection-related symptoms. According to studies, elderberry can shorten the length and intensity of cold and flu symptoms. Elderberry is a safe and natural remedy that can be used to enhance resistance to viral threats without the risk of harmful side effects associated with conventional treatments.
According to research, elderberry has broad spectrum antiviral action, which means it can stop a wide range of viruses from replicating. Elderberry is an affordable treatment that is widely available at most health food stores and is simple to include in a balanced diet.

According to research, elderberries have anti-inflammatory qualities that may assist to lessen inflammation brought on by viral infections. Elderberry has been demonstrated to provide advantages for respiratory health, including lowering airway inflammation and enhancing lung function.
Popular plant licorice has been used for many years to treat a wide range of illnesses, including viral infections. It is known for its immune-boosting and antiviral properties. We will explore licorice's antiviral properties and potential advantages in this essay.

Numerous substances found in licorice have been demonstrated to have antiviral effects. The most well-known of these compounds is glycyrrhizin, which has been shown to inhibit the replication of a variety of viruses, including influenza, HIV, and herpes simplex virus.

Glycyrrhizin works by interfering with the replication of the virus. This is accomplished by blocking the synthesis of viral RNA and DNA, preventing the assembly of new viral particles, and preventing the virus from entering host cells.

There are a number of possible advantages for licorice as an antiviral. Some of these benefits include:
It has been demonstrated that licorice improves immunological function, which can aid the body in warding off viral illnesses. Interferon, a protein that aids in controlling the immune response and reducing inflammation, is stimulated during this process.

It has been demonstrated that licorice lessens the intensity and persistence of viral infection-related symptoms. Licorice helps lessen the duration and intensity of cold and flu symptoms, according to studies. Licorice has been shown to possess anti-inflammatory qualities, which can help to reduce inflammation associated with viral infections. It has been demonstrated that licorice has broad-spectrum antiviral activity, which means that it can prevent the growth of numerous viruses.
Without the risk of the negative side effects associated with conventional therapies, licorice is a secure and natural therapy that may be used to improve resistance to viral threats.

It has been demonstrated that licorice provides digestive health advantages, including lowering gut inflammation and enhancing gut function. Licorice has been demonstrated to have positive effects on cardiovascular health, including lowering blood vessel inflammation and enhancing blood flow.

The medicinal herb andrographis, commonly referred to as "King of Bitters," has been used for ages in traditional medicine to cure a variety of ailments. It is indigenous to South Asian nations such as India, Sri Lanka, and Pakistan. Due to its antiviral, anti-inflammatory, and immune-stimulating characteristics, it has been utilized in Ayurvedic and Chinese medicine.

Andrographis contains various active compounds, including andrographolide, deoxyandrographolide, and neoandrographolide, which have been shown to have a wide range of pharmacological activities, including anti-inflammatory, antipyretic, and immunomodulatory effects. These substances have also been demonstrated to have antiviral activity against a variety of viruses, including the coronavirus, HIV, herpes simplex virus, influenza A and B, and HIV.

Andrographis has antiviral characteristics primarily as a result of its capacity to prevent viral reproduction in host cells. It has been demonstrated that andrographolide prevents the virus from attaching to the receptor on the host cell by binding to the viral surface protein. Andrographolide has also been demonstrated to prevent viral genes from being expressed and the creation of viral particles in infected cells.

Additionally proven to have immune-stimulating qualities, andrographis may strengthen the body's built-in defenses against viral infections. It has been shown to stimulate the production of white blood cells, including macrophages and natural killer cells, which are involved in the recognition and destruction of viral particles. Furthermore, andrographis promotes the synthesis of cytokines, such as interferons, which are essential for the immune system's defense against viral infections.

Andrographis has been proven to have antiviral, immune-boosting, anti-inflammatory, and antioxidant characteristics. These traits may help lessen the intensity of viral infection-related symptoms. Interleukin-6 and tumor necrosis factor-alpha, two pro-inflammatory cytokines that are frequently raised in viral infections and support the development of inflammation and tissue damage, have been demonstrated to be inhibited by it. Numerous conditions, such as respiratory infections, fever, sore throat, and diarrhea, have been treated with andrographis. It has been demonstrated to be beneficial in minimizing the severity and duration of symptoms brought on by upper respiratory tract infections, such as the common cold and flu. Andrographis has also been shown to be effective in treating viral hepatitis, herpes simplex virus infections, and HIV.
The safety profile of andrographis is among its most notable advantages. Traditional medicine has used it for decades without experiencing any negative side effects. High doses of andrographis, it is crucial to remember, have the potential to upset the stomach and result in nausea, vomiting, and diarrhea.

Different forms of administration and dosage guidelines

Popular herbal remedy echinacea is used for enhancing the immune system. Tablets, capsules, tinctures, and teas are just a few of the several forms it comes in. The suggested dosage is determined by the method of administration, the patient's age, health status, and other variables.

The most popular methods of administration for echinacea are tablets and capsules. They come in a variety of doses and intensities, usually weighing between 200 and 1000 mg per serving. The suggested dosage is determined on the patient's age and state of health. For adults, the typical dosage is 300-500 mg, three times a day, while for children, it is recommended to use half of the adult dosage. It is preferable to take echinacea capsules with food to increase absorption.

Echinacea is steeped in alcohol and water to make tinctures. They come in different strengths and dosages, usually ranging from 1:1 to 1:5, with the latter being the strongest. The strength of the tincture and the patient's health condition determine the suggested dosage of echinacea. The average dosage for a 1:1 tincture is 2-4 mL, three times day, whereas the suggested dosage for a 1:5 tincture is 0.4-1 mL, three times daily. It is best to consume echinacea tincture diluted in water, juice, or tea.

The plant is steeped in hot water to make echinacea tea. They are offered as loose leaf or tea bags. The recommended dosage of Echinacea tea depends on the strength of the tea and the individual's health status. The dosage for a standard potency tea is 1-2 cups, two to three times each day. One cup, two to three times a day, is advised for a stronger tea. You should drink echinacea tea hot or warm, with or without honey or lemon.

When using echinacea, it is crucial to adhere to the dosage recommendations in order to prevent side effects. Echinacea taken in high dosages can make you feel queasy, nauseous, and dizzy. In order to prevent becoming tolerant to the effects of echinacea, it is also advised against using it regularly for longer than eight weeks. Before consuming echinacea, anyone who are pregnant, breastfeeding, or have autoimmune problems should talk to their doctor.

A well-known herb with medical uses dating back hundreds of years is garlic. It is known to possess antibacterial, antifungal, and antiviral properties, making it an effective treatment for various health conditions. Although it is frequently used in cooking, there are a number of therapeutic uses for garlic as well.

Garlic is available in various forms for medicinal use. The most common forms of administration include:

The most potent form of garlic is raw garlic since it has all of the active ingredients that give it its therapeutic benefits. You can add chopped raw garlic to food or eat it raw, crush it, or both. Raw garlic has a strong flavor and smell, therefore some individuals might choose to consume it in another way.

There are several types of garlic supplements, including capsules, pills, and oils. These supplements are standardized to include a certain level of allicin, the key ingredient in garlic that gives it its therapeutic benefits. Garlic supplements are an excellent option for those who do not like the taste and odor of raw garlic.

Garlic is fermented for a long time—up to 20 months—to produce aged garlic extract. This procedure results in a milder garlic flavor and odor as well as an increase in the amount of specific active chemicals in garlic. Aged garlic extract is offered as liquid, pills, and capsules.

Macerating garlic in oil—typically olive or sunflower oil—creates garlic oil. Using this method, the active ingredients in garlic are extracted to create a concentrated oil that can be ingested or applied topically. Those who dislike the flavor and smell of raw garlic have a great alternative in garlic oil.

It is possible for the recommended amount of garlic to change depending not just on the method of administration but also on the ailment that is being treated. The following is a list of the recommended serving sizes for the various types of garlic:

The recommended dosage of raw garlic is one to two cloves per day, crushed or chopped and added to food. Consuming raw garlic on an empty stomach puts unnecessary strain on the digestive system and is therefore not recommended.

It's possible that different concentrations of allicin in garlic supplements will result in different dosage recommendations. The normal daily dosage ranges from 600 to 1200 milligrams (mg), taken in two or three equal portions. It is absolutely necessary to adhere to the dosage instructions listed on the packaging of the supplement.

It's possible that the concentration of active components in aged garlic extract will dictate how much of the suggested dosage you take. The normal daily dosage ranges from 600 to 1200 milligrams (mg), taken in two or three equal portions. It is absolutely necessary to adhere to the dosage instructions listed on the packaging of the supplement.

It is possible for the recommended dosage of garlic oil to change depending on the amount of active components present in the oil. When used physically or consumed orally, a common dosage is from one to two tablespoons per day. It is essential to follow the dosage guidelines on the product label carefully.
Garlic is generally safe when taken in the recommended dosages. Nevertheless, it may induce adverse consequences in some individuals, including the following:
Gastrointestinal discomfort, including bloating, gas, and diarrhea. Bad breath and body odor. Allergic reactions, including rash and itching. Blood thinning, which may raise the risk of bleeding in individuals who are taking drugs that already thin the blood.

Before beginning to take garlic supplements, it is imperative to speak with a qualified medical professional, particularly if you are already on any medications or have a pre-existing medical condition. Garlic has the potential to interact negatively with a number of drugs, particularly those used to thin the blood, which could result in unwanted side effects.

Elderberry, also called Sambucus nigra, is a well-known herbal antiviral that can be used to increase one's resistance to the effects of viral infections. As a treatment for the common cold, influenza, and various other respiratory illnesses, it has a long history of use. Elderberries have a high concentration of antioxidants and are believed to strengthen the immune system. It is sold in a number of different preparations, including syrup, lozenges, candies, capsules, and even beverages. In this section, we will discuss the different forms of administration and dosage guidelines of Elderberry.

Elderberry syrup is the most typical form of administration. It is simple to ingest, and it may be found in a variety of different health food stores. In order to make elderberry syrup, first the elderberries are simmered in water, and then either honey or sugar is added to sweeten the concoction. During this procedure, the beneficial components found in the berries are extracted and concentrated into a syrup for consumption. Elderberry lozenges are another popular form of administration. They are easy to transport and provide a steady supply of the active ingredients, which are released over time. To make elderberry lozenges, elderberry extract is combined with other natural ingredients, including sweeteners and flavorings. Consuming this herbal antiviral in the form of elderberry candy is a delicious and entertaining way to do so. Elderberry extract, gelatin, and natural sweeteners are the three components that go into their production. Elderberry gummies are an excellent option for toddlers and adults who have trouble swallowing tablets or capsules.

Elderberry capsules are a convenient form of administration for those who prefer to avoid the sweeteners found in syrup or gummies. The elderberry extract that is contained in the capsules is very concentrated, and they are quite simple to consume. They are available in different strengths and dosages.

Elderberry tea is a traditional form of administration. It is created by steeping dried elderberries or elderberry flowers in boiling water. Elderberry tea is abundant in antioxidants and immune-boosting compounds.

The elderberry supplement dosage that is suggested to take is different for each person, taking into account factors such as their age and current state of health. Before beginning treatment with elderberry, it is crucial to either follow the suggested dosage guidelines provided by the manufacturer or see a healthcare expert.

The amount of elderberry syrup that an adult should consume on a daily basis is equal to one tablespoon (15 ml). Children can take half the adult dosage. In cases of acute viral infections, the recommended dosage may be increased to one tablespoon (15 ml) four times per day.

Elderberry lozenges should be taken as directed by the manufacturer. The recommended dosage is typically one lozenge every 2-3 hours.

Elderberry gummies should be taken as directed by the manufacturer. The recommended dosage is typically 1-2 gummies per day. Elderberry capsules should be taken as directed by the manufacturer. The recommended dosage is typically 500-1000 mg per day. Elderberry tea can be consumed several times a day. For each cup of hot water, 1-2 teaspoons (5–10 grams) of dried elderberries are advised.

It is crucial to remember that elderberry should not be taken in place of standard medical care. It is an additional treatment that can help the immune system respond better to viral infections. Before consuming elderberry, expectant or nursing women should speak with their healthcare professional. Before consuming elderberry, anyone with autoimmune disorders, diabetes, or allergies should also speak with a healthcare professional.

Since ancient times, licorice has been used as a common herbal medicine for a number of illnesses, such as coughs, colds, sore throats, and digestive problems. It has also gained popularity as a potent antiviral agent, particularly in the treatment and prevention of viral infections. Glycyrrhizin and flavonoids, two active substances found in licorice root, are thought to have antiviral characteristics.

The several forms of licorice include dried roots, tea, pills, tablets, and liquid extracts. Before selecting the ideal solution for your needs, it is crucial to understand how each type of administration differs from the others and what pros and factors each one offers.

Tea and decoctions are frequently made with dried licorice roots. The dried roots are cooked in water for several minutes to create tea, which is then drunk. The roots are boiled for a long time to extract the active ingredients in decoctions, a stronger type of tea. There are several places to get dried licorice roots, which are frequently used to create traditional medicines.

Licorice tea is an easy and convenient way to enjoy the benefits of licorice. Licorice roots are steeped in boiling water for several minutes to make the tea, which is then filtered and drunk. The dosage of licorice tea can be changed by steeping the roots for various amounts of time or by drinking more or less tea. It is frequently accessible at health food stores.

Additionally, pills and capsules of licorice are offered. These methods of administration offer a standardized amount of licorice extract and are practical and simple to take. In health food stores and online, capsules and pills can be found. The dosage should be taken as directed by the manufacturer.

Liquid extracts are another popular form of licorice administration. The licorice roots are cooked in either water or alcohol to create these extracts, which are then condensed and packaged. Liquid extracts are highly concentrated and should be taken according to the dosage instructions on the label. Important to be aware of is the alcohol content of some liquid extracts, which may not be acceptable for everyone.
The right amount of licorice to take depends on the person's age, health, and method of administration. Before beginning any herbal remedies, it is always best to speak with a trained healthcare professional to be sure they are secure and suitable for you.

The dosage for dried roots or tea depends on how potent the product is. The recommended daily intake is 1-2 cups of licorice tea or 2-4 grams of dried roots. It is important to remember that licorice tea shouldn't be drank in big amounts over an extended period of time because it could have negative effects.
Licorice extract is normally given in regulated doses via capsules and tablets. The suggested dosage varies according on the particular product, and it is essential to follow the manufacturer's instructions carefully. Generally speaking, it is advised to take 500–1,000 mg of licorice extract per day.
Liquid extracts offer licorice in a very concentrated form, so the dosage needs to be changed. It is advised to begin with a lesser dosage and raise it gradually as necessary.

Liquid extracts are often taken in doses of 2-4 mL per day, though this might vary depending on the product.

The medicinal herb andrographis has been used for many years to cure a variety of diseases in traditional medicine. It is currently renowned for having strong antiviral qualities that make it a useful natural treatment for viral illnesses. Andrographis is accessible in a number of forms, like as extracts, capsules, teas, and tinctures, each of which has specific dose requirements and techniques for administration.

A concentrated form of the herb known as andrographis is obtained through the extraction process. This extract is available in liquid form or as a powder, and it is often used in traditional medicine to treat various health conditions, including viral infections. The normal dosage of andrographis extract is between 300 and 500 mg per day, with smaller amounts being more frequently advised. It is typically taken with a meal to increase absorption, and it's crucial to stick to the manufacturer's dose recommendations.

With pre-measured quantities that may be used with water or another beverage, andrographis capsules are a practical way to take the herb. Depending on the severity of the infection, the person's weight, and their general health, the dosage for andrographis capsules is normally between 400 and 800 milligrams per day. To optimize absorption, capsules should be taken with food, and it's crucial to stick to the manufacturer's recommended dosage levels.

Andrographis tea is a popular way to take the herb, as it is easy to make and can be consumed throughout the day. Simply simmer one teaspoon of the dried herb in a cup of hot water for five to ten minutes, drain, and then drink to produce andrographis tea. The dosage for andrographis tea can be consumed up to three times each day.

The herb andrographis is extracted with alcohol or another solvent to produce andrographis tincture, a concentrated liquid version of the herb. Traditional medicine frequently employs this variety of andrographis to treat a range of ailments, including viral infections. The normal dosage of andrographis tincture is 10 to 20 drops per day, with smaller amounts being more effective. It is typically taken with a meal to increase absorption, and it's crucial to stick to the manufacturer's dose recommendations.
Depending on the delivery method, the level of infection, the patient's weight, and general health, the dosage of andrographis may change. Following the manufacturer's recommended dosage is crucial because taking too much andrographis can have adverse consequences like digestive trouble, headaches, and allergic reactions.
The recommended dosage of andrographis for adults is typically between 300 and 800 milligrams per day, depending on the form of administration. Andrographis should not be administered to minors under the supervision of a medical professional.

It's crucial to remember that andrographis shouldn't be taken for longer than two weeks at a time because prolonged use can have negative effects like headaches and upset stomachs. It's crucial to see your doctor before taking andrographis if you're expecting, nursing, or taking any medications.

Potential side effects and contraindications

The purple coneflower, often known as echinacea, is a popular herbal treatment with a number of health advantages, such as antiviral, anti-inflammatory, and immune-boosting characteristics. Prior to utilizing echinacea, it is crucial to be informed of any potential side effects and contraindications as with any drug or dietary supplement.

One of the most common side effects of Echinacea is allergic reactions, particularly in individuals who are allergic to plants in the daisy family, such as ragweed, chamomile, or marigolds. An allergic reaction may cause a skin rash, itching, swelling, and breathing problems. Stop using echinacea and get help right away if you have any of these symptoms.

After using echinacea, certain individuals may develop gastrointestinal upset, including nausea, diarrhea, and stomach pain. The majority of these adverse effects are minor, and they may disappear when taking Echinacea with food or at a lesser dosage. Nevertheless, it's crucial to stop using Echinacea and seek medical advice if these symptoms worsen or persist.

Immunosuppressants, corticosteroids, and pharmaceuticals used to treat autoimmune illnesses are among the drugs with which echinacea may interact. It is crucial to seek medical advice before using echinacea if you are currently using any of these medications.

There is limited information on the safety of Echinacea during pregnancy and breastfeeding. Therefore, it is advised that women who are expecting or nursing refrain from using Echinacea unless specifically instructed to do so by a medical expert.

Due to its immune-boosting qualities, Echinacea should be avoided by people with autoimmune diseases like lupus or rheumatoid arthritis. By boosting the immune system, echinacea might make these illnesses worse.

Rare cases of liver damage linked to echinacea use have been made. Abdominal pain, nausea, vomiting, and a yellowing of the skin or eyes are possible symptoms. If you suffer any of these symptoms, it's critical to stop using Echinacea and get help right once.

The common herb, garlic, which has a long history of use in both food and medicine, has been linked to a number of health advantages, including antiviral and antibacterial properties. Garlic may create adverse effects and interact with drugs or health problems, just like any other herbal product.
Gastrointestinal upset, including bloating, flatulence, and heartburn, is one of the most typical side effects of garlic. These effects are frequently attributed to garlic's high sulfur content, which can irritate the digestive tract. These adverse effects may be more common in people with sensitive stomachs or digestive diseases like irritable bowel syndrome (IBS).

Some people may experience skin rashes or allergic reactions from garlic. People who handle raw garlic or apply garlic oil topically have been known to experience contact dermatitis, a kind of skin inflammation. Symptoms may include redness, itching, and blistering.

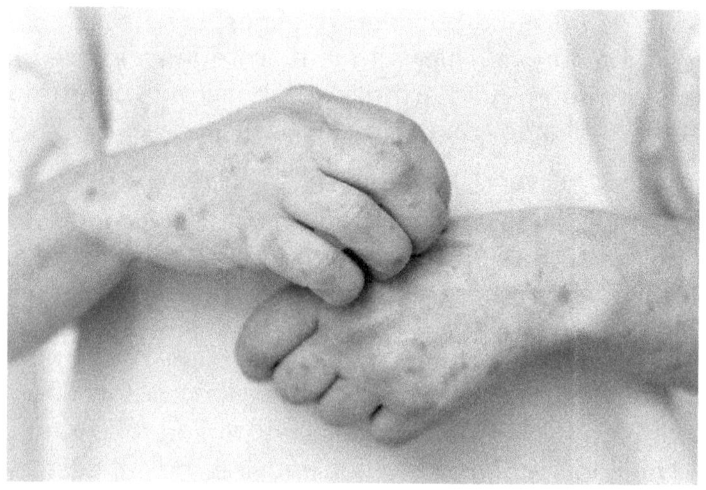

Because of garlic's well-known intense fragrance, eating a lot of it may cause poor breath and body odor. The release of volatile sulfur compounds from garlic, which can be expelled through the skin and breath, is what causes this effect.

Garlic has blood-thinning properties and may increase the chance of bleeding, especially when taken in excessive doses or together with other blood-thinning medications. Before using garlic supplements, individuals who are taking blood thinners like aspirin or warfarin should speak with their doctor.

Garlic may interact with a number of drugs, including several HIV treatments, blood thinners, and drugs that reduce blood pressure. Combining garlic supplements with certain drugs may raise the risk of bleeding or cause dangerously low blood pressure. If you are taking any drugs, it is crucial to speak with a healthcare professional before using garlic supplements.

When used in the authorized dosages, garlic supplements are generally regarded as safe for the majority of people.

However, there are some conditions in which using garlic is not advised, including:

People who have bleeding disorders should avoid taking supplements containing garlic because it could increase their risk of bleeding. Garlic supplements are not recommended for pregnant or breastfeeding women due to limited research on their safety. Before surgery or dental operations, garlic supplements should be avoided as they may increase the risk of bleeding.

Sambucus nigra, also known as elderberry, is a popular medicinal plant valued for its antiviral qualities. It has been used for millennia to treat colds, flu-like symptoms, and respiratory infections. Additionally, it is a well-liked nutritional supplement and a typical component of over-the-counter cold and flu medications. Like any other herb or medication, it is usually thought to be safe, but it is still vital to be aware of any potential side effects and contraindications.

Although elderberry is usually thought to be harmless, some people may experience some adverse effects. The gastrointestinal symptoms include nausea, vomiting, and diarrhea are the most frequent adverse effects. These side effects are usually mild and self-limited, but in some cases, they can be severe.
Elderberry can also cause allergic reactions in some people. Itching, hives, swelling, and breathing difficulties are a few of the mild to severe allergic reaction symptoms. Elderberries can cause allergic reactions, so anyone experiencing one should get help right away.

Blood sugar levels may be reduced by elderberry, which is another potential negative effect. People with diabetes who use drugs that also lower blood sugar levels may find this to be of concern. Diabetes patients should utilize elderberry with caution and have their blood sugar levels closely checked.

In addition, elderberry can interact with certain medications. For instance, it can weaken the effects of immunosuppressant drugs and strengthen the effects of diuretic drugs. Before taking elderberry, it's crucial to discuss your prescription use with your doctor.

Elderberry is generally considered safe for most people, but there are some individuals who should not take it. These include:

It is advised to avoid elderberry because there is not enough data on its safety during pregnancy and breast-feeding. Elderberries may increase immune system activity, which can be harmful for those who suffer from autoimmune conditions like lupus, rheumatoid arthritis, and multiple sclerosis.

Elderberry can drop blood pressure and blood sugar levels, thus those with hypotension, hypoglycemia, or other illnesses that impact blood pressure or blood sugar levels should use it with caution.

Although elderberry syrup is a well-known natural treatment for children's colds and flu, it should not be administered to infants under the age of one due to the possibility of botulism.

The medicinal herb licorice, also known as Glycyrrhiza glabra, has been utilized for thousands of years in traditional medicine for its multiple health advantages. Licorice root contains many active compounds, including glycyrrhizin, flavonoids, and saponins, that are believed to contribute to its therapeutic effects. Licorice has been utilized for the treatment of a broad variety of health ailments, including those related to the digestive and respiratory systems, as well as for its ability to reduce inflammation and fight viruses. Licorice, like all other herbal treatments, may have side effects and interact negatively with certain drugs. However, licorice is less likely to induce adverse reactions than other herbal remedies.

Consuming licorice can lead to an increase in blood pressure, which is one of the most prevalent negative effects of doing so. Glycyrrhizin, which is found in licorice root, is a chemical that can cause the body to retain sodium and water, which can ultimately contribute to an elevation in blood pressure. The consumption of substantial quantities of licorice over a protracted period of time is the most likely to bring about this effect. Hypokalemia, often known as low potassium levels, is another potential adverse consequence that might arise from taking significant amounts of licorice. This is because glycyrrhizin can interfere with the body's ability to regulate potassium levels, leading to potentially serious health problems.

The levels of various hormones in the body can also be affected by licorice root, particularly the hormone cortisol. Increased levels of the hormone cortisol, which helps the body respond to stress, can be caused by excessive consumption of licorice. This can result in a variety of symptoms, including weight gain, mood swings, and high blood pressure.

Consumption of licorice can also lead to gastrointestinal issues, such as nausea, vomiting, and diarrhea. This is especially true when high amounts of licorice are ingested over an extended length of time or for a prolonged period of time.

Since licorice is a plant, just like any other plant, it has the potential to give certain people allergic reactions. It is necessary to be aware of the symptoms of an allergic reaction, which include swelling of the face, lips, or tongue; hives; and difficulty breathing. Since allergic reactions to licorice are uncommon, but they can be dangerous, it is important to be aware of the symptoms of an allergic reaction.

Licorice root should be avoided during pregnancy and breastfeeding, as it can interfere with hormonal balance and may have adverse effects on fetal development. Licorice can cause an increase in blood pressure, thus people who already have high blood pressure or heart disease should avoid it or consume it in moderation at the very most.

Because licorice root has the potential to mess with one's blood sugar levels, diabetics are strongly advised to abstain from taking licorice or to do so only under the supervision of a trained medical practitioner. Consuming licorice root can have an effect on kidney function; therefore, people who already have kidney disease should avoid doing so.

Corticosteroids, diuretics, and several medicines used to treat heart disease are among the medicines that potentially interact with licorice root. It can also lessen the effectiveness of birth control tablets and worsen the side effects of drugs used to treat high blood pressure.

Andrographis is a herb that has long been utilized in Ayurvedic medicine. Because of its bitter flavor, it is often referred to as the "king of bitters." Andrographis has been studied extensively for its medicinal properties, especially its antiviral effects. It has been demonstrated to have antipyretic, anti-inflammatory, and antioxidant qualities, as well as positive benefits on the immune system. But like all herbs, andrographis has the potential to produce negative side effects and may not be suitable for everyone.

When used at the proper doses, andrographis is usually regarded as safe, however some people may develop side effects. The most common side effects of Andrographis include:

Andrographis can lead to digestive problems like diarrhea, bloating, and discomfort in the abdomen. These adverse effects are typically manageable by lowering the dose or stopping use.

Some people may experience headaches after taking Andrographis. This adverse effect is typically modest and disappears on its own over time.

In rare cases, Andrographis can cause an allergic reaction. Itching, hives, or swelling of the face, lips, tongue, or throat may be symptoms of an allergic reaction. Other symptoms may include anaphylaxis. Seek medical attention immediately if you experience any of these symptoms.

Because it is known to bring blood pressure down, andrographis should not be taken by those who are currently taking hypertension medication. There is not enough information available to evaluate whether or not andrographis is safe to use during pregnancy or while breastfeeding. It is best to avoid Andrographis during these times.

Andrographis should not be taken by patients who are currently being treated for certain medical illnesses or who are taking particular drugs. Some contraindications of Andrographis include:

Andrographis may have the ability to stimulate the immune system, which may make the symptoms of autoimmune disorders such as multiple sclerosis, lupus, and rheumatoid arthritis worse.

Andrographis may make persons more likely to bleed, particularly those who already have a bleeding disease or who are using blood-thinning medication. Because it may raise the risk of bleeding both during and after surgical procedures, andrographis should be discontinued at least two weeks before the scheduled operation.

Andrographis may lower blood sugar levels, so it should be used with caution in individuals with diabetes who are taking medication to lower their blood sugar.

Because andrographis has the potential to stimulate the immune system, it should not be taken in conjunction with immunosuppressant medicine. Doing so could compromise the efficacy of the immunosuppressant treatment.

CHAPTER IV

Herbal Antiviral Recipes and Remedies

Herbal antiviral teas, tinctures, syrups, and other remedy recipes

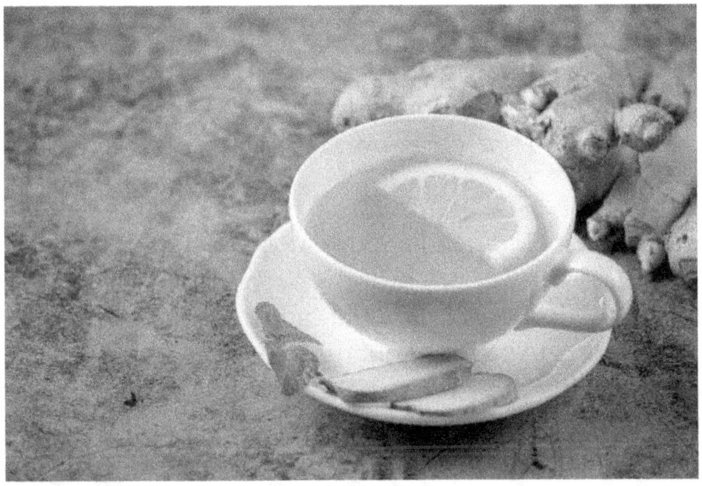

Herbal antivirals are non-pharmaceutical therapies that are derived from plants and have the potential to either treat or prevent viral infections. Teas, tinctures, syrups, and other medicinal concoctions are only some of the many ways that herbal antivirals can be prepared and taken in the body. In this section, we will talk about a variety of herbal antiviral remedies and the benefits that they offer.

Boosting one's immune system and warding off viral infections can be accomplished by regularly drinking herbal antiviral teas, which are simple to make and can be consumed whenever desired. Here are some popular herbal antiviral tea recipes:

Echinacea is a well-known herb for its ability to stimulate the immune system, and echinacea tea is a popular way to consume this herb. To prepare echinacea tea, add 1 teaspoon of dried echinacea root or 2 teaspoons of dried echinacea leaves to a cup of boiling water. After allowing it to steep for 10–15 minutes, drain it before consuming. Ginger is another potent herb that has antiviral qualities, and it may be found in ginger tea. To prepare ginger tea, thinly slice some fresh ginger root and put it in a cup of water that is already boiling. Before ingesting, allow it to soak for five to ten minutes, then strain it. Honey or lemon juice are two other options for enhancing the flavor.

Elderberry has been studied for its ability to fight viruses and reduce inflammation, and elderberry tea is a popular way to consume this fruit. To create elderberry tea, combine one to two teaspoons of dried elderberries with one cup of water that has been brought to a boil. After allowing it to steep for 10–15 minutes, drain it before consuming.

Tea made from licorice has been shown to help increase immune function due to the licorice root's antimicrobial and anti-inflammatory characteristics. To create licorice tea, combine one to two tablespoons of dried licorice root with one cup of water that has been brought to a boil. After allowing it to infuse for 10–15 minutes, drain it before consuming.

Herbal tinctures are liquid extracts of herbs that are typically taken orally. They are a concentrated form of the herb that are typically produced by soaking the herb in alcohol or vinegar for a period of time before using it. Here are some herbal antiviral tincture recipes:

Garlic has powerful antiviral effects and can be utilized to help the immune system fight off infections. To prepare a garlic tincture, finely cut some fresh garlic and place it in a jar. Pour enough alcohol or vinegar over the garlic to cover it, then set it aside for two weeks to six weeks to ferment. After straining the liquid, put it in a dark bottle and put it away.

Andrographis is a powerful antiviral plant that can both aid in the prevention of viral infections and treat those that have already occurred. To prepare a tincture of andrographis, finely chop some fresh leaves of the plant and place them in a bottle. Pour enough alcohol or vinegar over the leaves to cover them, then let the mixture sit for two weeks to six weeks. After straining the liquid, put it in a dark bottle and put it away.

Olive leaf has antiviral and immune-boosting properties. To prepare olive leaf tincture, finely chop some fresh olive leaves and place them in a jar with some alcohol. Pour enough alcohol or vinegar over the leaves to cover them, then let the mixture sit for two weeks to six weeks. After straining the liquid, put it in a dark bottle and put it away.

Antiviral herbal syrups are delicious medicines that can be administered to prevent or treat viral infections. These syrups are sweet and made from herbs. All age groups are able to safely consume them because they often consist of honey or another naturally occurring sweetener. Here are some herbal antiviral syrup recipes:

Elderberry is a well-known herbal treatment for viral infections, and taking this plant in the form of elderberry syrup is a manner that is both delicious and effective to do so. In a saucepan, mix together one cup of dried elderberries, three cups of water, one cinnamon stick, and four cloves to make elderberry syrup. After bringing the mixture to a boil, reduce the heat and continue to simmer for thirty to forty minutes. After you have strained the liquid, add one cup of honey and stir it until it is completely dissolved. Bottle the syrup and store in the refrigerator.

Ginger is a potent plant that can help reduce inflammation and combat viruses, which in turn can help the immune system function more effectively and ward against diseases. In a saucepan, mix together one cup of chopped fresh ginger, four cups of water, and two cups of sugar to produce ginger syrup. Bring the mixture to a boil, then lower the heat and continue to simmer for thirty to forty minutes. After straining the mixture, bottle it up and put it in the refrigerator to chill.

Root licorice is an effective antiviral and immune-boosting plant that can be used to assist in the battle against infections. In a sauce pan, mix together one cup of chopped licorice root, four cups of water, and two cups of honey to make licorice syrup. Bring the mixture to a boil, then lower the heat and continue to simmer for thirty to forty minutes. After straining the mixture, bottle it up and put it in the refrigerator to chill.

Andrographis is a potent antiviral plant that has been demonstrated to help fight off a range of illnesses. It has been used for this purpose for a long time. In a sauce pan, combine one cup of dried andrographis, four cups of water, and two cups of honey to make andrographis syrup. Bring the mixture to a boil, then lower the heat and continue to simmer for thirty to forty minutes. After straining the mixture, bottle it up and put it in the refrigerator to chill.

The herb cinnamon is known for its warming and antibacterial properties, making it useful for warding off illnesses and bolstering the immune system. In a pot, combine one cup of cinnamon chips or cinnamon sticks, four cups of water, and two cups of sugar to produce cinnamon syrup. Bring the mixture to a boil, then lower the heat and continue to simmer for thirty to forty minutes. After straining the mixture, bottle it up and put it in the refrigerator to chill.

Since ancient times, people have turned to herbal medicine to treat a wide range of conditions, including viral infections. In recent years, there has been a rise in interest in natural medicines, and more individuals are turning to herbs for help in preventing and treating illnesses caused by viruses. In this section, we will go over a variety of herbal antiviral medicines that may be manufactured in the comfort of one's own home.

Honey and cinnamon are two components that have been widely recognized for their ability to inhibit the growth of bacteria and viruses. They have antiviral properties, and when blended in a tea, they can help ease sore throats and fight off viral infections. To prepare a cup of honey and cinnamon tea, simply bring one cup of water to a boil, stir in one teaspoon of cinnamon powder, and then let the mixture simmer for a few minutes. Then, add a teaspoon of honey and stir. If you want the finest benefits, drink this tea two or three times every day.

Both ginger and lemon are well-known for their ability to strengthen one's immune system, especially when combined. Ginger contains gingerols and shogaols, which have anti-inflammatory and antiviral effects. Vitamin C, which can be found in abundance in lemon, is absolutely important for maintaining a strong immune system. To prepare ginger and lemon tea, bring one cup of water to a boil, add a few slices of fresh ginger, and then let the mixture soak for a few minutes. After that, add the juice of half a lemon to the tea and whisk it up. If you want the finest benefits, drink this tea two or three times every day.

A spice known as turmeric has a long history of application in various forms of alternative medicine. Curcumin, a component of this spice, possesses anti-inflammatory, antioxidant, and antiviral qualities, and it is responsible for the spice's yellow color. Piperine, a component found in black pepper, facilitates the body's uptake of curcumin and is one of the pepper's many health benefits. To prepare a cup of tea with turmeric and black pepper, simply bring one cup of water to a boil, stir in one teaspoon of turmeric powder, and then let the mixture steep for a few minutes. Then, add a pinch of black pepper and stir. If you want the finest benefits, drink this tea two or three times every day.

Dosage guidelines for each remedy

Depending on how the herb is prepared, different dosages of Echinacea tea are advised. The typical dosage for dried Echinacea root or herb is 1-2 grams steeped in boiling water for 10-15 minutes, up to three times a day. The suggested dosage for fresh Echinacea is 3–4 grams steeped in boiling water for 10–15 minutes, up to three times daily.

One to two grams of fresh or dried ginger, soaked in boiling water for ten to fifteen minutes, can be consumed up to three times daily. It's crucial to keep in mind that ginger may interfere with specific drugs and shouldn't be used in large amounts while pregnant.

Elderberry tea can be taken up to three times day with 1-2 tablespoons of dried elderberries boiled in boiling water for 10-15 minutes. It's vital to remember that elderberries should not be taken uncooked due to their toxicity. Elderberry tea shouldn't be consumed constantly for longer than five days.
Licorice tea can be had up to three times daily with 1-2 grams of dried licorice root steeped in boiling water for 10-15 minutes. It's crucial to remember that licorice shouldn't be consumed constantly for longer than 4 weeks and may interfere with some drugs.

Depending on the tincture's potency and the user's state of health, different amounts of garlic tincture are advised. Garlic tincture can be taken up to three times per day, diluted in water or juice, at doses of 2-4 mL (or 40-80 drops). In order to prevent gastrointestinal discomfort and other side effects, it is crucial to start with a low dose and gradually raise it over time.

Andrographis tincture can be taken up to three times per day, diluted in water or juice, at doses of 1-3 mL (or 20–60 drops). In order to prevent gastrointestinal discomfort and other side effects, it is crucial to start with a low dose and gradually raise it over time.

Depending on the tincture's potency and the user's state of health, different dosages of olive leaf tincture are advised. For olive leaf tincture, the usual dosage range is 2-4 mL (or 40–80 drops) up to three times daily, diluted in water or juice.

Adults are normally advised to have 1-2 teaspoons of elderberry syrup 2-3 times per day, while children over 1 are advised to consume 1/2-1 teaspoon. Elderberry syrup should not be given to infants under 1 year old.

It is typically recommended to take 1-2 teaspoons of ginger syrup 2-3 times per day for adults and 1/2-1 teaspoon for children over the age of 1. Ginger syrup should not be given to infants under 1 year old.

It is typically recommended to take 1-2 teaspoons of licorice syrup 2-3 times per day for adults and 1/2-1 teaspoon for children over the age of 1. Licorice syrup should not be given to infants under 1 year old.

It is typically recommended to take 1-2 teaspoons of Andrographis syrup 2-3 times per day for adults and 1/2-1 teaspoon for children over the age of 1. Andrographis syrup should not be given to infants under 1 year old.

It is typically recommended to take 1-2 teaspoons of cinnamon syrup 2-3 times per day for adults and 1/2-1 teaspoon for children over the age of 1. Cinnamon syrup should not be given to infants under 1 year old.

The dosage for Honey and Cinnamon tea is typically one to two cups per day, as needed. However, it is important to note that honey should not be given to children under one year of age due to the risk of botulism.

One to two cups of ginger and lemon tea should be consumed daily, as needed. Individuals with gallstones or blood issues should avoid ginger because it may interact with some drugs.

One to two glasses of the turmeric and black pepper tea should be consumed daily, as needed. It is crucial to remember that turmeric could interact with several drugs, such as blood thinners and diabetes treatments.

Tips for making and storing herbal remedies

Since ancient times, individuals have turned to herbal medicine to treat a wide range of conditions, including viral infections. In spite of the fact that there are a great deal of useful herbs and cures, it is essential to ensure both their efficacy and safety by correctly preparing and storing them. In this section, we will go over some suggestions for the preparation and storage of herbal treatments.

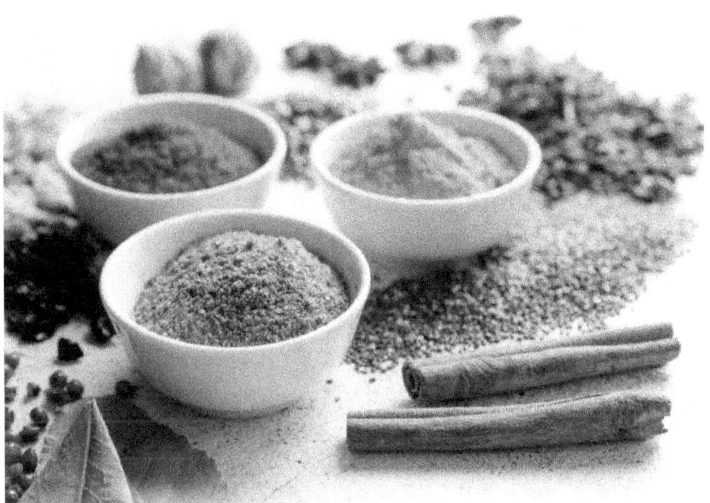

The quality of the herbs used in herbal remedies is of utmost importance. It is recommended that you choose herbs that are fresh and organic. Herbs that have been around for a long time or that have been incorrectly preserved are likely to have lost some of their effectiveness and may not be as effective as they once were. It is essential to acquire herbs from a reliable supplier in order to ensure that they are of the highest possible quality and purity.

Teas, tinctures, syrups, and capsules are just few of the forms of herbal medicine that can be prepared using the many different ways available. Each approach has a unique set of benefits and drawbacks, and selecting a method may be contingent on the particular herb being utilized as well as the effects that are intended. It is critical to conduct adequate research and adhere to correct preparation procedures in order to get the intended outcomes.

When preparing tea, it is essential to use the appropriate proportion of herbs to water and to steep the herbs for the appropriate amount of time in order to extract the therapeutic qualities of the herbs. For making tinctures, the herbs are soaked in alcohol or vinegar to extract their medicinal properties, and the strength of the tincture can be adjusted by varying the ratio of herbs to liquid. To make a concentrated syrup that can be added to drinks or taken by the spoonful, herbs are simmered in water while a sweetener such as honey or sugar is added. Herbal supplements can be taken in the form of capsules, which can either be filled with powdered herbs or liquid extracts of the herbs.

It is crucial to store herbal remedies in the correct manner in order to keep their effectiveness and safety intact. To stop the development of mold and preserve the freshness of herbs, they should be kept in a dark, dry area away from direct sunlight and any kind of moisture. It is recommended to store herbs in airtight containers, such as glass jars or bags, to prevent oxidation and loss of essential oils. This can be accomplished by removing oxygen from the container.

There is a possibility that herbal treatments, especially tinctures and syrups, have a shelf life that must be respected. It's important to label the remedies with the date of preparation and to discard any that have expired or show signs of spoilage.

Even though herbal medicines are usually risk-free, it is essential to use extreme caution and strictly adhere to the dosing instructions in order to prevent any unwanted consequences. Some herbs may have an adverse reaction when combined with certain drugs or may not be suitable for use by specific groups of people, such as children or pregnant women. Before beginning treatment with any herbal remedy, it is important to discuss your medical history and prescription regimen with a trained medical professional. This is especially important if you already have a pre-existing ailment.

When preparing herbal remedies, it is imperative that correct hygiene procedures be adhered to in order to eliminate the risk of contamination and guarantee the products' viability. Before working with herbs or preparing medicines, make sure to wash your hands and use clean tools, containers, and work surfaces. Also make sure to scrub your nails. To further protect against the spread of bacteria, it is recommended that you make use of distilled water or water that has been previously boiled and allowed to cool.

To guarantee the efficacy of herbal treatments while also ensuring their safety, quality assurance tests should be performed on a routine basis. This may include testing the herbs for purity and potency, monitoring the expiration dates of prepared remedies, and regularly reviewing and updating preparation methods and dosage guidelines.

CHAPTER V

Building Resilience with Lifestyle Changes and Natural Support

How altering one's lifestyle might strengthen immunity and prepare one for viral threats

Our body is protected from potentially hazardous pathogens like viruses, bacteria, and fungus by our immune system, which is responsible for its function. However, the immune system is susceptible to being compromised by a variety of conditions, including stress, poor nutrition, insufficient sleep, and lack of physical activity. For this reason, it is absolutely necessary to maintain a healthy lifestyle that supports and develops the immune system in order to guard against the effects of viral infections. In this section, we will explain how making adjustments to one's lifestyle can strengthen one's immune system and build resilience against the effects of viral infections.

Maintaining a strong immune system requires a diet that is both nutritious and balanced. Consuming a wide variety of fruits, vegetables, whole grains, and lean sources of protein can supply the required nutrients and antioxidants to enhance immunological function. For example, vitamin C, found in citrus fruits and leafy greens, has been shown to enhance immune function and reduce the severity of respiratory infections. Zinc, which is essential for immune function and may be found in seafood, nuts, and seeds, is especially vital for people who are getting older. Because they can cause inflammation and make the immune system less effective, foods that have been processed and that are heavy in fat should be consumed in moderation.

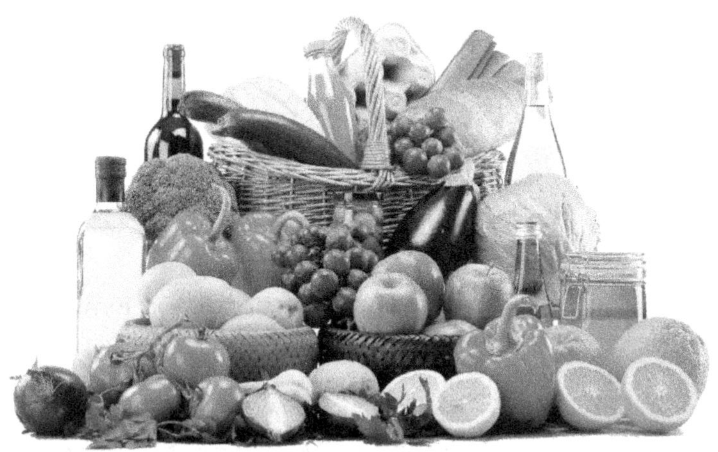

Maintaining a strong immune system requires adequate sleep. When we sleep, our bodies create cytokines, which are proteins that play an important role in the body's defense against infection and inflammation. A lack of sleep can result in a reduction in the synthesis of cytokines, which can make an individual more susceptible to infection. It is recommended that children and teenagers receive even more sleep than the minimum of 7-9 hours per night, while adults should get at least that much.

Through the processes of boosting circulation and improving lymphatic flow, physical activity can improve immune function. Exercise has been shown to enhance the production and activity of immune cells, such as natural killer cells and T cells, which can help fight infections. It is advised that individuals get at least 150 minutes of exercise per week at a moderate intensity, or 75 minutes of exercise per week at a vigorous intensity.

The production of cortisol, a hormone that inhibits immunological function, can be increased in response to stress, which can have the effect of making the immune system less effective. As a result, it is essential to investigate and experiment with various methods of stress management, such as yoga, deep breathing, meditation, and other relaxation practices. Participating in activities such as hobbies, visiting with loved ones, and engaging in physical activity all have the potential to assist in the reduction of stress.

It's crucial to stay hydrated to keep your immune system strong. Dehydration can cause a reduction in lymphatic flow, which in turn can have an effect on the function of the immune system. It is advised that individuals consume at least 8 cups of water every day, and even more during times of intense physical activity or when the weather is particularly hot or humid.

Smoking can weaken the immune system by damaging the cilia in the respiratory tract, which can impair the body's ability to remove pathogens. In a similar vein, drinking an excessive amount of alcohol can suppress the development of immune cells, which in turn can impair the immune system. Giving up smoking and cutting back on alcohol use are two lifestyle changes that can improve immune function and lower the likelihood of acquiring a viral illness.

Advice on how to get more restful sleep, manage stress, and fit exercise into your daily schedule

In order to maintain a robust immune system and increase one's resistance to viral assaults, it is essential to prioritize getting sufficient amounts of sleep, managing one's stress levels, and including routine physical activity as part of one's daily routine. In order to assist you in leading a lifestyle that is more healthy and well-balanced, the purpose of this section is to discuss methods for enhancing the quality of your sleep, lowering your levels of stress, and introducing physical activity into your daily routine.

It is necessary to get adequate sleep in order to maintain general health and wellness, including the operation of the immune system. Here are some tips for improving your sleep quality:

Keeping the same schedule for when you go to bed and when you get up each day can help regulate the body's natural sleep-wake cycle, making it easier to get to sleep and allowing you to feel more refreshed when you get up.

Getting into the habit of doing something soothing before bed can send a message to your body that it's time to wind down and get ready for sleep. This may involve engaging in activities such as taking a relaxing bath, reading a book, or engaging in relaxation practices such as meditation or taking slow, deep breaths.

Your ability to fall asleep and stay asleep can be significantly influenced by the surroundings of your bedroom. In order to establish an atmosphere that is conducive to sleep, ensure that your room is dark, cool, and quiet. Investing in supportive bedding as well as a comfortable mattress can also help enhance the quality of sleep.

It may be more difficult to fall asleep after engaging in activities that stimulate the mind, such as using technological gadgets or watching exciting television shows. Make it a point to steer clear of these activities at least one hour before going to bed.

Both caffeine and alcohol are known to interfere with normal sleep patterns and to diminish the quality of sleep. Reduce the amount of these things that you consume, particularly in the hours coming up to your bedtime. Long-term stress can have a detrimental effect not just on one's physical health but also on their mental health and their immune function. Here are some tips for reducing stress in your life:

If you are able to identify the factors that contribute to the stress in your life, you will be in a better position to develop efficient coping mechanisms. Activities that help alleviate stress and promote relaxation, such as yoga, meditating, and deep breathing, are examples of such activities.

Having a sense of social support and lowering stress levels are both benefits that may be gained by spending time with friends and family. Spending time on things that bring you pleasure, like reading, listening to music, or participating in a hobby, can help lower stress levels and increase general well-being.

Seeking the assistance of a mental health professional can be beneficial if you are having trouble dealing with the effects of stress on your own.

Participating in regular physical activity can assist boost immunological function as well as general health. The following is a list of suggestions for incorporating physical activity into your everyday routine:

If you've never worked out before, it's best to begin with goals that are easily attainable and gradually build up both the intensity and the length of your exercises as time goes on. Engaging in activities that you enjoy can make it easier to stick with an exercise routine over the long-term.

It is important to set goals for your fitness regimen that are both reasonable and challenging in order to maintain your motivation and achieve success. Increasing your total level of physical activity can be accomplished by the completion of simple tasks, such as using the stairs rather than the elevator or walking rather than driving. You may help keep yourself accountable and motivated by working out with a workout partner, enrolling in an exercise class, or participating in an exercise club.

In conclusion, adopting adjustments to your lifestyle to increase the amount of sleep you get, decrease the amount of stress you experience, and increase the amount of exercise you do can support a strong immune system and create resilience against viral threats. You may improve your general health and well-being by following these steps, which will work to do so in the near term as well as over the course of the longer term.

Overview of other natural supports for the immune system

Our body's immune system acts as the primary line of defense against harmful pathogens such as illnesses and

infections. It is made up of an intricate web of cells, tissues, and organs that cooperate to defend the body against pathogenic germs including parasites, viruses, and bacteria. It is essential to keep one's immune system in good shape in order to ward off illness and assist the body in its fight against infections. A healthy immune system can be supported and strengthened in a variety of ways, including through the utilization of natural therapies and supplements. The following is a rundown of some of the most powerful naturally occurring immune
system boosters:

Vitamin C is an effective anti-oxidant that contributes significantly to the proper functioning of the immune system. It helps to stimulate the the production of white blood cells, which are tasked with battling infections and are produced as a result of this stimulation. Citrus fruits, berries, kiwis, papaya, broccoli, spinach, and tomatoes are examples of foods that contain a significant amount of vitamin C.

It is impossible for the immune system to operate effectively without enough vitamin D levels. It not only improves the immune cells' ability to ward against infections, but it also helps to control the overall generation of immune cells. Sun exposure is the best source of vitamin D, but it can also be found in fatty fish, fortified dairy products, and supplements.

Zinc is a mineral that is important for immune function. It helps to stimulate the production of white blood cells and also plays a role in the development of antibodies. Foods that are rich in zinc include oysters, beef, pork, chicken, beans, and nuts.

Probiotics are good bacteria that reside in the gut and enhance immune system health. They help to maintain a healthy balance of gut bacteria and also enhance the production of antibodies. Probiotics are foods that have been fermented, including yogurt and kefir kimchi, and sauerkraut, as well as in supplements.

Adaptogenic herbs are a group of herbs that help the body to cope with stress and promote balance in the body. Some adaptogenic herbs that support the immune system include ashwagandha, rhodiola, and astragalus.
Essential oils are highly concentrated plant extracts that can help to boost the immune system. Some essential oils that are known for their immune-supporting properties include eucalyptus, tea tree, peppermint, and lemon.
Green tea has a high concentration of antioxidants and also contains chemicals that have qualities that are beneficial to the immune system. It does this by helping to increase the development of immune cells, which in turn improves those cells' ability to fight off infections.

Exercise is an important way to support immune function. It assists in the reduction of inflammation, enhancement of circulation, and stimulation of the creation of white blood cells. In addition, consistent physical activity can help to alleviate stress and promote better sleep, both of which are critical for optimal immune function.
Getting adequate sleep is important for immune function. During the time that we are asleep, our bodies create cytokines, which are proteins that play an important role in the body's defense against infection and inflammation. Lack of sleep over an extended period of time can have the effect of suppressing immune function and making the body more susceptible to illnesses.

Immune system performance might be negatively impacted by chronic stress. Finding strategies to reduce stress, like through yoga, deep breathing, or meditation, can assist the immune system and improve general health.

It is essential to keep in mind that natural supports for the immune system, despite the fact that they may be beneficial, should in no way be used in place of medical therapy or guidance. It is essential that you get medical help as soon as possible if you notice any symptoms that could indicate an infection or disease. If you have a pre-existing medical condition or are already on medication, it is extremely important to discuss the use of any dietary supplements or herbal remedies with a qualified medical professional before beginning their use.

CHAPTER VI

Herbal Antivirals for Specific Viral Threats

Overview of the most efficient herbal antivirals for fighting various viral threats

Humans can be exposed to a wide variety of viral dangers, each of which calls for a different strategy to be taken in terms of treatment and prevention. Herbal antivirals have seen a surge in popularity in recent years as an effective alternative to conventional antiviral medication for the treatment of viral infections. In this section, we will discuss some of the most common viral threats and the herbal antivirals that have been found to be effective against them.

The influenza virus is the primary cause of influenza, more often known as the flu. Influenza is a respiratory ailment that is highly contagious. Fever, cough, sore throat, aches and pains in the muscles, and weariness are some of the symptoms. The influenza virus can be passed from person to person either through the air we breathe or by coming into contact with infected objects or surfaces.

Elderberry, echinacea, and ginger are examples of potent herbal antivirals that have been demonstrated to be useful against the flu. Elderberry has been proven to block the capacity of the influenza virus to enter host cells, which in turn reduces the intensity of flu symptoms and shortens their duration. It has been discovered that echinacea can stimulate the formation of white blood cells in the body, which can assist in the battle against the virus. It has been shown that ginger can lessen the intensity of flu symptoms due to the antiviral and anti- inflammatory qualities it possesses.

The herpes simplex virus (HSV) is the source of the viral infection known as herpes. There are two types of herpes: oral herpes, which causes cold sores on or around the mouth, and genital herpes, which causes sores in the genital area. Herpes is a condition that is considered to be chronic since it can recur at any time during a person's life.

Licorice root and lemon balm are two examples of herbs that have been demonstrated to have antiviral properties and be useful against herpes. It has been discovered that the licorice root contains a substance known as glycyrrhizin, which is capable of preventing the herpes virus from replicating. It has been shown that the herb lemon balm, which contains antiviral characteristics, can lower both the frequency and severity of herpes outbreaks.

The human papillomavirus, sometimes known as HPV, is a virus that is spread through sexual contact and has been linked to both genital warts and cervical cancer. In addition to the larynx, the anus, and the penis, the virus is also capable of causing cancer in other regions of the body.

Green tea and astragalus are two examples of herbs that have been identified as having antiviral properties that are beneficial against HPV. Catechins, which are found in green tea, have been demonstrated to reduce the risk of contracting the HPV virus by preventing its replication.

Astragalus has been found to stimulate the immune system and may help the body fight off the virus.

The immune system is weakened and the body has a harder time fighting off other diseases as a result of the human immunodeficiency virus, also known as HIV. If treatment is not received, acquired immunodeficiency syndrome (AIDS), which is caused by HIV, can develop.

Garlic and St. John's wort are two examples of efficient herbal antivirals that have been studied for their potential to combat HIV. Allicin, which is found in garlic, is a compound that has been demonstrated to inhibit the reproduction of the HIV virus. Garlic is often used as a treatment for HIV. It has been shown that taking St. John's wort can reduce the amount of HIV in a person's body.
Viral infections that affect the liver include hepatitis B, C, and CHepatitis B. The hepatitis B virus can spread when contaminated blood or other bodily fluids are touched, whereas the hepatitis C virus is transmitted almost exclusively through contact with infected blood.

Herbal antivirals that have been found to be effective against hepatitis B and C include milk thistle and licorice root. Milk thistle includes a component known as silymarin that has been proved to protect the liver and minimize inflammation produced by hepatitis viruses. These benefits have been demonstrated through research. Researchers have discovered that licorice root possesses antiviral characteristics and that these properties may assist the body in fighting against hepatitis infections.

Dosage guidelines and potential side effects for each herbal antiviral

As individuals search for alternate methods to prevent and treat viral infections, the use of herbal antivirals has become an increasingly common practice. Although these treatments are not known to pose any significant health risks, it is essential to familiarize oneself with the correct dosing instructions for each herb and to be aware of any potential adverse effects.

Echinacea can be taken as a tea, tincture, or capsule. To make echinacea tea, soak one to two teaspoons of dried echinacea root or leaves in one cup of boiling water for ten to fifteen minutes, and then sip the tea up to three times daily. To use the tincture, take between 2 and 4 milliliters (mL) three times day. For the capsules, take 300-500 mg three times a day. Rarely, a person could experience side effects such as an upset stomach, dizziness, or a rash on their skin. Echinacea should be avoided by individuals who are hypersensitive to plants belonging to the daisy family.

Garlic can be consumed in raw, cooked, or supplement form. Chopped raw garlic can be added to foods, or it can be used as a dietary supplement in the form of capsules or tablets. The daily amount of garlic supplements that should be taken is between 600 and 1,200 mg. The use of garlic is typically regarded as harmless, although eating too much of it might lead to digestive issues and poor breath. Before using garlic supplements, people who are already on medications that thin the blood should discuss this with their doctor.

Elderberry can be taken as a tea, syrup, or capsule. Elderberry tea can be prepared by steeping one to two tablespoons of dried elderberries in one cup of boiling water for ten to fifteen minutes. The tea can be consumed up to three times per day. The recommended serving size for the syrup is one tablespoon (15 mL) four times per day. For the capsules, take 500 mg three times a day. Side effects may include mild upset stomach and diarrhea. Consuming high amounts of elderberry can lead to hazardous effects, so this fruit should be avoided whenever possible.

Licorice can be consumed as a tea, capsule, or extract. To make licorice root tea, soak one to two teaspoons of dried licorice root in one cup of boiling water for ten to fifteen minutes. The tea can be had as often as three times a day. Take between 200 and 400 milligrams of the capsules three times a day. Take between 250 and 500 milligrams of the extract three times a day. Those who have high blood pressure or kidney disease should avoid consuming licorice. A prolonged use could result in a potassium deficiency in addition to other adverse consequences.

Andrographis can be taken as a capsule or tablet. The recommended dosage is 400-800 mg twice a day. Side effects may include digestive upset, headache, and fatigue. Andrographis may interact with certain medications, including blood thinners, so it is important to consult with a healthcare provider before using.

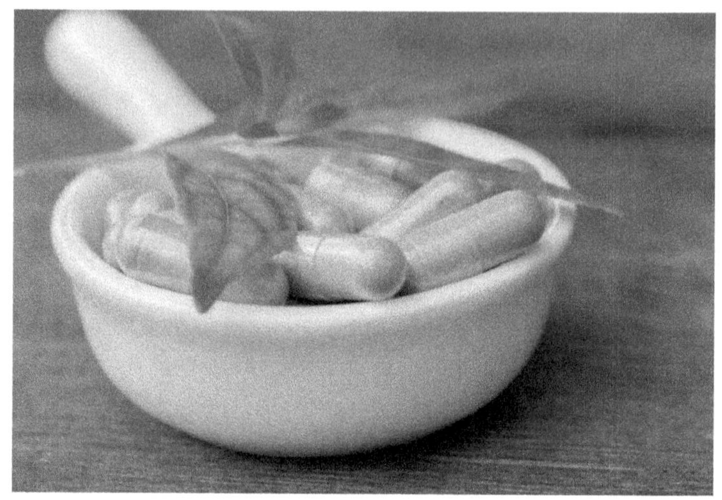

Olive leaf can be ingested in the form of a tea, a pill, or an extract. To make olive leaf tea, soak one to two tablespoons of dried olive leaves in one cup of boiling water for ten to fifteen minutes, and then sip the tea up to three times daily. For the capsules, take 500-1,000 mg twice a day. For the extract, take 500-1,000 mg twice a day. Olive leaf is regarded safe to consume in most cases; nevertheless, excessive consumption might lead to gastric discomfort.

It is essential to keep in mind that the correct dosage as well as the potential adverse effects may change depending on variables such as age, current health status, and the other medications that are being used at the same time. Before beginning treatment with any new herbal cure, it is important that you discuss your condition with a healthcare professional. In addition, it is essential to get herbal supplements from reliable sources in order to make certain that they are both pure and effective.

CONCLUSION

Recap of the book's main points and how herbal antivirals can help build resilience against viral threats

Throughout this book, we have explored the world of herbal antivirals and how they can be used to support the immune system and help the body defend against viral threats. We have covered the many classes of herbal antivirals, their characteristics, and the potential advantages they may offer, as well as their recommended dosages and any possible adverse reactions that may occur. In addition, we have investigated the use of herbal antivirals in conjunction with conventional treatments, as well as the utilization of other naturally occurring immune system boosters, in order to strengthen resistance to viral assaults.

The necessity of understanding the immune system and how it functions to protect against viral infections is one of the primary points that can be gained from reading this e-book. The immune system is an intricate network that consists of cells, tissues, and organs that cooperate with one another to recognize and destroy harmful organisms. When we have a better understanding of how the immune system functions, we are better able to take measures to support it and build up our resistance against viral threats.

Herbal antivirals are a powerful tool in supporting the immune system and helping the body fight off viral infections. Echinacea, garlic, elderberry, licorice, and andrographis are just a few examples of potent herbal antivirals that can be used to support the immune system. It is essential to adhere to the dosage guidelines and be aware of any potential adverse effects when using any of these herbs because each one possesses distinctive qualities and may provide potential advantages.

In addition to antivirals made from herbs, there are additional naturally occurring supports for the immune system that have the potential to be helpful. Maintaining a strong and healthy immune system requires a combination of lifestyle factors, including lowering stress levels, engaging in regular physical activity, and eating a nutritious diet.

Additionally, it is essential that we have a solid understanding of the particular viral dangers that may harm us as well as the herbal antivirals that are the most successful against those dangers. Elderberry, for instance, has been proven to be effective against the influenza virus, and andrographis has been used to treat dengue fever and a variety of other tropical disorders.

Overall, the use of herbal antivirals can be a valuable tool in building resilience against viral threats. If we are able to gain a grasp of the characteristics and possible benefits of these herbs, as well as the recommended dosages for them and any possible adverse reactions to them, we will be able to include them into our health routines in a way that is both safe and beneficial. It is possible for us to establish robust immune systems and better defend ourselves against viral threats by combining herbal antivirals with other natural supports for the immune system as well as conventional treatments when these are necessary.

Final thoughts and a call to action to strengthen your immune system and defend against viral threats.

As we get to the end of this e-book, it is essential to keep in mind that the development of a strong immune system is absolutely necessary in order to guard against the dangers posed by viral infections. We have gone through the several ways in which herbal antivirals might strengthen our immune system, including their qualities, applications, and possible advantages. We have also discussed the different forms of administration and dosage guidelines for each herbal remedy.

Modifications to our lifestyles, such as increasing the amount of sleep we get, decreasing the amount of stress we allow ourselves to experience, and increasing the amount of physical activity we do, are examples of the natural immune system boosters that we have addressed in addition to antiviral herbs. In addition to that, we have gone over particular virus dangers and the herbal antivirals that are the most powerful against them.
It is essential to keep in mind that herbal antivirals, despite the fact that they have the potential to be an effective instrument in constructing resistance against viral dangers, should not be relied on exclusively. It is essential to adhere, where necessary, to the recommendations and treatments of traditional medical professionals, particularly in the case of serious infections.
The use of herbal antivirals as part of our regular routine can be an important preventative measure that we can take to strengthen our immune systems and better defend ourselves against viral infections. Nevertheless, it is essential to do so under the supervision of a qualified

medical expert and to be aware of the potential adverse effects and indications not to use the treatment.

Finally, it is important to remember that building a strong immune system and protecting against viral threats is a continuous process. It takes dedication and effort to sustain a healthy lifestyle, including the incorporation of natural supports and seeking medical assistance when it is essential.

We strongly encourage readers to take measures to strengthen their immune systems and protect themselves from the dangers posed by viral infections. Making even minor adjustments to the habits we follow on a daily basis can have a considerable impact on the overall health and well-being we experience. On this path toward optimal health, we hope that this e-book has been helpful in providing both information and direction, and we thank you for reading it.

Thank you for buying and reading/ listening to our book. If you found this book useful/ helpful please take a few minutes and leave a review on the platform where you purchased our book. Your feedback matters greatly to us.